Michael, Amy, Brandon, Ariana

Stay Healthy.

Jeff

IT'S A GREAT TIME TO BE A PHYSICIAN

Building a Healthcare System that Works

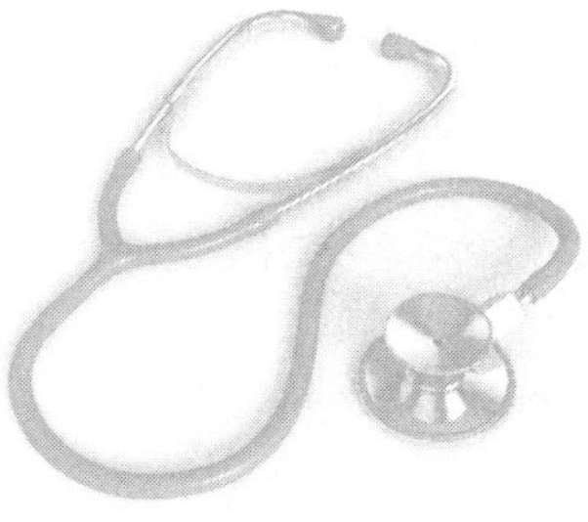

Jeffrey A. Weisz, MD

with

Susan Albers Mohrman

and

Arienne McCracken

IT'S A GREAT TIME TO BE A PHYSICIAN:
Building a Healthcare System that Works

Second River Healthcare Press
26 Shawnee Way, Suite C
Bozeman, MT 59715

Phone (406) 586-8775
FAX (406) 586-5672

Editor: Tiffany L. Young
Cover Design: Lan Weisberger – Design Solutions
Cover Art: Roger Schillerstrom
Typesetting/Composition: Neuhaus/Tyrrell Graphic Design

Weisz, Jeffrey, Mohrman, Susan Albers, McCracken, Arienne
IT'S A GREAT TIME TO BE A PHYSICIAN:
Building a Healthcare System that Works / Jeffrey Weisz, MD,
with Susan Albers Mohrman & Arienne McCracken

ISBN-13: 978-1-936406-14-2 (hardcover)
ISBN-13: 978-1-936406-15-9 (softcover)
ISBN-13: 978-1-936406-16-6 (e-book)

1. Physician Leadership 2. Innovative Healthcare 3. Patient Centered Care

Library of Congress Control Number: 2012942801

First Printing January 2013

Table of Contents

Dedicated to patients
and their care providers everywhere.

Foreword

This book by Dr. Jeffrey A. Weisz, current executive medical director of the Northwest Permanente Medical Group and former executive medical director of the Southern California Permanente Medical Group (SCPMG), is a modern "Rosetta Stone" for health system leaders and health policy scholars. Just as the actual Rosetta Stone, uncovered in 1801 by one of Napoleon's soldiers, revealed the previously hidden mysteries of Egypt, so *It's a Great Time to Be a Physician: Building a Healthcare System That Works* uncovers for the reader the details of the inner workings of one of largest and most successful physician-led integrated healthcare systems in the country. Although interesting enough in itself, this tour through the myriad elements of what has made the SCPMG so successful is all the more significant because it comes at a time when the nation is in need of many more such care systems but woefully ignorant about how to create them.

The nation faces a healthcare cost and quality crisis that, unresolved, threatens the stability of the US economy and the fabric of social justice upon which our society ultimately rests. The Patient Protection and Affordable Care Act of 2010 (PPACA, more recently shortened to Affordable Care Act or ACA), despite the current political rancor it has created, has set the nation on a course to cover many more Americans than have previously had access to healthcare services. But the experience Massachusetts has had with similar legislation shows that increased coverage without concomitant changes to how healthcare services are organized and paid for can "break the bank" of government, businesses, and individuals. Because of this risk, Blue Cross Blue Shield of Massachusetts has embarked on the "Alternative Quality Contract" project to foster the integration of care delivery into systems paid by a "global payment" or capitation. Similarly, PPACA called for a new form of provider entity, the Accountable Care Organization (ACO), to be created and fostered by the Medicare program and paid for improvements in quality and costs. Many more ACOs are currently being created by payers and providers in the "commercial" (non-Medicare) market. These changes in the structure of care delivery and payment are usually referred to as "delivery system reform," and are probably the last best hope to address the quality and cost crisis we face.

Delivery system reform faces many obstacles including: entrenched vested interests in the status quo, the costs and risks inherent in changes of this magnitude, potential public and political resistance, legal and regulatory barriers and the temptation to believe that this is just one more idea whose time will pass. But perhaps the biggest obstacle to change is simply the general absence of "know-how" to create and manage this transformation. During the mid- to late 1990s some similar changes were envisioned, leading to the creation of Integrated Delivery Systems and Physician-Hospital Organizations, many of which ultimately failed. One major reason for these failures was the *naïveté* with which physicians and hospitals created these new organizations. Many entered into capitation or other risk-bearing contacts with payers without the organizational leadership, governance and management tools to make them successful. The same thing could happen again. But it should not. Because fifteen years later there are many more successful models for new emerging delivery systems to emulate. SCPMG and the other Permanente Medical Groups are just such systems.

In this book Dr. Weisz lays out eight essential capabilities that any aspiring medical group, integrated delivery system or ACO must have in place to succeed. Each is vital, but none stands on its own. All eight need to be combined in a synergy that drives the organization toward its mission. Last addressed (but first in importance in my mind) is effective physician leadership. Physicians drive of the majority of quality outcomes and at least 80 percent of medical costs. Effective physician leadership requires both personal qualities and a receptive organizational culture. Effective leaders must have followers. Physicians are not reflexive followers. They will become so if they believe in the mission of the organization, participate in its governance and are supported in those aspects of clinical autonomy that lead to high quality care and a fulfilling career. This creates the fertile ground for applying the tools that Dr. Weisz details.

Prepayment for services through capitation, global payment or the like creates the incentive to keep patients well, not profit from illness. Thus, prevention, early detection and the management of chronic diseases become the lynchpins of the organization, aligning the interests of patients and physicians in a way that fee-for-service payments do not. This creates the group focus on the welfare and satisfaction of each individual in a population of patients served, not just the sick ones, and is the basis for patient-centered care. This "group responsibility" leads directly to the notion of teamwork, not just among physicians but between physicians and staff, and between physicians and administrators. The team approach which characterizes Kaiser Permanente has smoothed otherwise difficult tasks, such as the implementation of system-wide electronic medical records, the acceptance of objective clinical goals with accompanying measurement and transparency, the application of evidence-based practice, the systemization of clinical care pathways, and the amalgamation of all these tools to create a culture of constant innovation and improvement. This is the pathway to the future for American medicine.

It is my fervent hope that the lessons Dr. Weisz has presented in this book become a "playbook" for developing ACOs and other physician-led delivery systems. That said, the accomplishments of SCPMG, other Permanente Medical Groups and other medical group-based organizations such as the Geisinger Health System, the Mayo Clinic, the Henry Ford Health system and others are not easily won. Success requires a dedication to a new sense of mission; courageous leadership not afraid to fail or to overcome the skepticism and even wrath of colleagues; cooperation with non-physician executives such as hospital administrators and payers; and an abiding patience and will. But the history of SCPMG and other such heroic organizations are a living testament to what is possible, and this book should help lead the way to making the Permanente experience one that can be shared across the country, for the betterment of patient care and the evolution of a more satisfying environment for medical practice. Good work, Dr. Weisz.

Francis J. Crosson, MD
Director of Public Policy
The Permanente Medical Group

Preface

My purpose in writing this book is to open up conversations among physicians about how they can take charge of their destiny and participate in creating high-value healthcare. I strongly believe that we need to be leaders in shaping both how healthcare reform unfolds and the new healthcare system that will address the challenges faced today in an era of limited resources and escalating demand. I believe that we can build a win-win system; one where high-quality care is delivered at affordable prices, and where physicians are fairly compensated while experiencing the satisfaction and pride of professional accomplishment and contribution. I believe this because we have been building such a system in the Southern California Region of Kaiser Permanente (KPSC).*

Imagine mediocre service and patients who gritted their teeth when they had to deal with a large, confusing healthcare system. Imagine excellent doctors, nurses and staff, delivering good quality and technical care, but who were sometimes embarrassed to admit where they worked. KPSC wasn't known to be a great healthcare delivery system, and certainly not one that was focused on the patient experience. In the year 2000, our promise to be a system that was focused on prevention remained unfulfilled.

I'm sure our millions of members were happy to know that they received good care at an affordable price, but that doesn't mean that they felt their needs were being met in the best possible way.† In fact as recently as 2005, many, including our local *Los Angeles Times*, declared that HMOs were, at best, "in unstable condition" with "members bolt[ing] to other plans," because they wanted more choices and more flexible plans.[1]

** The Kaiser Permanente Medical Group Program primarily consists of three cooperating entities: Kaiser Foundation Health Plan, Inc. and its health plan subsidiaries ("Health Plans"), Kaiser Foundation Hospitals, and the Permanente Medical Groups. The Permanente Medical Groups are independent medical groups. The Health Plans and Kaiser Foundation Hospitals are not-for-profit corporations that engage in charitable, educational, and research activities, including the provision and arrangement of health care. The relationship between each Health Plan and its Medical Group counterpart is established through an annual contract in which the Medical Group is compensated primarily on a fixed amount per member per month. Each Medical Group is solely responsible for determining how its physicians are compensated from the amounts received by the Medical Group. When I mention "KPSC" (Kaiser Permanente Southern California) in this book, I am referring to the three cooperating entities in Southern California as we work together.*

† People who sign up for healthcare through Kaiser Permanente are referred to as "members."

That was the past. Today I can proudly say that KPSC has come a very long way. It has responded to the changing healthcare environment and introduced a variety of health plan products to better address the needs of employers to share costs with employees and to introduce more flexibility for members. But new health plan products and new payment systems are not what have propelled us forward. We introduced fundamental change in the way we utilize our resources to deliver care and have truly focused on our mission of prevention and keeping people healthy.

We are now a world-class healthcare system that attracts top physicians, nurses, pharmacists, and a whole host of healthcare providers from universities around the world. Our patients receive excellent care, plain and simple, and we are proud of the service we provide. Southern California Permanente Medical Group (SCPMG) has hired fifteen hundred new physicians since 2004. We are now among the national leaders in areas including breast cancer and colon cancer screenings, hypertension control, osteoporotic fracture reduction, the use of an electronic medical record (EMR) in our outpatient and inpatient delivery system, and in diabetes certification of primary care physicians. Our robotic surgery program now leads the nation in patient safety, outcomes, and cost efficiency. Based upon the vast amount of data generated by our EMR and disease registries, we regularly contribute to the medical literature. Since 2000, membership in KPSC has grown from 3 to 3.5 million. It is projected to reach 4.5 million by 2019. Our patient satisfaction surveys and other metrics show how far we have come. Our Consumer Assessment of Healthcare Providers and Systems (CAHPS) healthcare rating has improved from below the national seventy-fifth percentile in 2008 to above the ninetieth percentile in 2011. Consumer Assessment of Health Providers and Systems Hospital Survey (HCAHPS) reports that KPSC's hospitals are now collectively performing at or above the seventy-fifth percentile in inpatient hospital service, up from the fiftieth percentile in 2008. Our goal is to move to the ninetieth percentile. We continue to search for ways to improve.

Why should you care? Because when I look at today's US healthcare system as a whole, I'm disheartened at what I see. Uncoordinated care, overutilization of expensive tests, drugs, and procedures, underutilization of preventive measures, a focus on illness, and insufficient attention paid to patient safety both in and out of the hospital are just a few of the problems that are pervasive and entrenched in American healthcare today. Commonwealth Fund studies consistently put US healthcare toward the bottom of the pack for outcomes such as longevity, efficiency, access, and safety, although we spend twice as much per capita on healthcare than any other country.[2]

Our country desperately needs an affordable, high-quality healthcare system, and a healthier population. Many economists see these two goals as essential to determining the health of our economy and to the vigor of our society in years to come. The simultaneous demand for quality care, improved outcomes, and value is increasingly central to the healthcare debate. The focus of healthcare reform (such as the Affordable Care Act) includes such things as electronic medical records, data transparency with measurable outcomes, greater accountability, more effective coordination of healthcare, tireless attention to building evidence-based medical care processes that work, and greater value for healthcare dollars spent. These, plus a relentless focus on prevention and on putting the patient front and center, have guided our journey to excellence at KPSC.

I'm writing this book for my fellow physicians, whose voices haven't been sufficiently heard in all the din of healthcare reform in the last few years. We bemoan "what is happening to American healthcare" and the resulting impact on how we "have to" practice medicine. We can do better than that. We are a profession full of extremely well-educated, competent professionals, who can do remarkable things to heal and cure patients. Shame on us if we don't become part of the solution to the challenges facing healthcare rather than seeing ourselves as victims. This book is a call to action.

I believe that it is precisely because there is so much change in the air that this is truly a great time to be a physician. If we step up to the plate, we can help develop healthcare approaches that work for our patients, our economy, and us. I've seen the physicians at SCPMG rise to this challenge, and from this I've learned a lot about how physicians can and must shape healthcare.

We physicians have access to amazing new medical capabilities. We also have information technologies that enable each provider to have unprecedented information about patients to underpin our care decisions. We can lead the way in making sure that our medical systems are designed to yield the levels of performance needed and expected by our society. We need to help shape the healthcare system of the future—to make sure that we are not overwhelmed by cost escalation and the increased demand stemming from changing demographics, unhealthy lifestyles, limited resources, uneven quality of care, and poor access. We need to identify ways to use resources more effectively and efficiently, and to develop integrated healthcare processes that avoid redundancy, inefficiency, undetected risk factors, and patient safety threats. Our practice patterns must focus not narrowly on creating the conditions for each of us as individuals to develop and apply our technical acumen, but widely, to enable the overall system to more effectively use resources to promote health and treat illness.

In short, we have to travel the same course as so many sectors of our economy that have found that they have to do more with less. To do so they've had to get out of their comfort zones and deliver greater value. We have to understand that value is in the eyes of the consumers and the payers of our services, not in our own self-assessment of whether we're delivering great care.

The healthcare landscape changes when we physicians find our voices and channel our passion for medicine into creating better approaches. I have been fortunate to head SCPMG during a time of great opportunity: a time when the national leadership of Kaiser Permanente committed KP to becoming a healthcare leader for the world. I'm proud that SCPMG and Kaiser Foundation Hospitals and Health Plan are rising to meet the challenge. I have worked with a tireless, talented, and committed team of physician leaders who have relished the opportunity to build a healthcare system to promote wellness and excellence. They have inspired physicians throughout the region to become actively engaged in building greatness. Our physicians have not passively waited for the latest edict to come down from above to tell them what to do.

American healthcare's journey will be long and arduous, and there's no denying that the lives of many physicians will change. In fact, they've already changed, but not necessarily in ways that physicians shaped, nor that we feel are working to ensure high-quality and enhanced outcomes. In this book I've chronicled what I have learned about how medical practice changes as a system learns to deliver high-value to patients and society. Young physicians coming out of medical school should expect an ever-changing landscape, to work as part of an integrated team, and should be prepared to continually improve the systems they work in. In this book, I have identified the eight trends that I believe are strongly impacting the practice of medicine, and what the implications are for physicians. This includes providing checklists at the end of the chapters so that physicians can reflect on their own practices and the extent to which they are adapting to these trends. An additional purpose is to allow young physicians to think about the kind of setting in which they choose to practice medicine, and the leadership roles that lie ahead.

From now on, value will be defined as how well we keep people healthy, not just how well we treat them when they are ill. We will become comfortable with the transparency and exposure as well as the incredible power of integrated care made possible by the EMR. We will continually change as we incorporate the rapidly emerging evidence about efficacy and best practice. We will get used to being paid for performance. Patients will come to us better informed, with a clearer sense of how they want to approach their own medical care, and we will have to incorporate their expectations. Most importantly, we have a responsibility to have a loud and clear voice in shaping the change that is certain to characterize healthcare in the future. We need to make sure the changes lead to high-quality, patient-focused care, improved outcomes, and higher value. We will have to step up and lead.

So take a look at the following chapters and consider the trends that are described. Also consider what KPSC—yes, that funny capitation system you thought had nothing to offer you—has done. Our journey is far from complete, but it is well underway. Physicians are leading our transformation, and in doing so, we're learning how to work collaboratively with the many stakeholders in our system. Our approaches and our solutions are powerful and applicable to many other systems. The integrated nature of our system has provided an extraordinary opportunity to put in place new approaches —accountable care, medical homes, integrated care pathways, wellness and prevention, telemedicine, outcomes-based rewards, and evidence-based medicine—that are the elements of most reform efforts today. As you read this book, you'll be reading about the elements of the healthcare system of the future, as well as your role in it.

The book describes general trends in healthcare, and expresses my point of view about how physicians can leverage their capabilities to create far more effective healthcare for society. It draws on the stories of many extraordinary physicians across the Southern California region as we have addressed these trends with the express purpose of creating a high-value healthcare system. Becoming a great healthcare system is a prodigious effort. Many, many people have made KPSC the success story that it is, and this book is all about them.

Our entire SCPMG executive team has worked tirelessly and collaboratively to build an infrastructure that has enabled profound change in our value formula and in our outcomes. I have been privileged to lead this extraordinary leadership team. Throughout this change we've shared the work, been excited by each other's ideas, and had each other's backs when the going got rough. My leadership team was composed of Dr. Michael Kanter, regional medical director of Quality and Clinical Analysis; Dr. Paul Minardi, regional medical director of Operations; Marilyn Owsley, business administrator of Finance, Systems, and Contracts; Dr. Jeffrey Selevan, medical director of Business Management; and Tom Williamson, business administrator of Operations.

SCPMG is a physician partnership, and I have worked with a truly gifted and supportive SCPMG Board of Directors. An amazing staff of regional leaders has contributed to our various initiatives. I have been continuously impressed by and thankful for the deep expertise, strong leadership, and unflagging energies of our regional chiefs of service. Together with the area chiefs of service, they have risen to the challenge of identifying important domains where KPSC would become a national leader. I am also indebted to the area medical directors, medical group administrators, and a host of other leaders in the thirteen medical centers and areas that constitute the Southern California Region of Kaiser Permanente. Throughout the book you will see references to these people who have achieved so much by enlisting the support of people throughout the region, and by getting change to happen.

It is important to note that over six thousand physicians comprise SCPMG. They make it the outstanding healthcare partnership it is today. As I move to my next leadership position as executive medical director of the Northwest region of KP, I will miss this remarkable group of physicians.

In this book I have highlighted the leadership role that physicians and SCPMG have played. But our physician partnership is one element of a larger enterprise, and our transformation has been occurring in tandem with the Health Plan and Hospital system of Kaiser Permanente. I have been especially blessed to have as my partner Dr. Ben Chu, president, Southern California Region, Kaiser Foundation Health Plan, Inc. & Hospitals, and to collaborate with John August, the executive director of the Coalition of Kaiser Permanente Unions. George Halvorson, the chairman and chief executive officer of Kaiser Permanente, Bernard Tyson, the president and COO of Kaiser Permanente, and Dr. Jack Cochran, the executive director of the Permanente Federation, have set the tone throughout the entire Kaiser Permanente system for striving to achieve excellence and leadership in healthcare.

A special thanks goes to Noreen Schob, my executive assistant, who has worked with me since I became executive medical director in 2004. Noreen is a wonderful, dedicated assistant who has worked tirelessly supporting me and the patients of Kaiser Permanente.

I'd also like to thank Jerry Pogue of Second River Healthcare Press. As the publisher of this book, Jerry offered valuable feedback and ideas. His knowledge of the healthcare industry and insight about publishing for the healthcare audience helped us refine and hone these chapters.

Dr. Sue Mohrman and Arienne McCracken wrote this book with me. It has truly been a team effort. I have appreciated their energy and skills in gathering information to illustrate the fundamental changes that are occurring in healthcare throughout the country. They also worked to spotlight case information about what we have been doing at KPSC to fundamentally change our system and about the role our physicians have played in this transformation. They have been instrumental in translating my heartfelt beliefs about what's important in the practice of medicine.

I am indebted to my wife, Carolyn, who has supported me and my career at SCPMG.

Thank you, Dad, for encouraging me to become a physician. If I had to do it again, I would still follow your recommendations.

Jeffrey A. Weisz, MD
Executive Medical Director,
Southern California Permanente Medical Group
January 1, 2004 – December 31, 2011

President and Executive Medical Director,
Northwest Permanente
January 1, 2012 – present

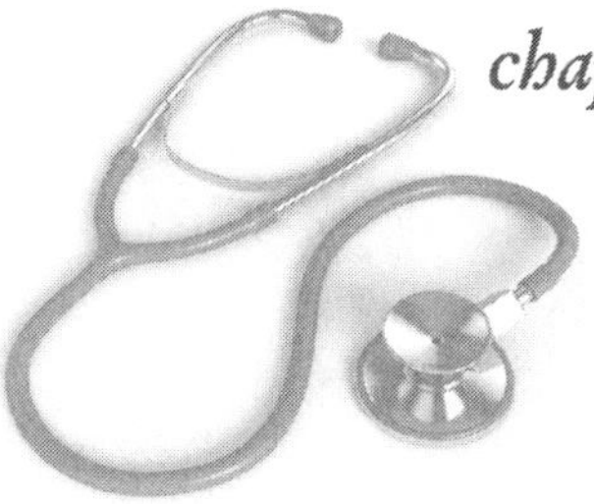

chapter one

An Exciting Time to Be a Physician

It's a great time to be a physician! We are in the middle of momentous changes that can make this profession even more satisfying and rewarding.

Is this a good time to be a physician? Absolutely! In fact, there has never been a better time. Let me tell you why. We are in the midst of significant changes in healthcare—changes that will help us be more effective clinicians. These changes will enable us to better accomplish what we were trained to do in medical school—to care for and improve the health and well-being of our patients, and to uphold the Hippocratic Oath.

I'm taking down my shingle and going home. It's a terrible time to be a physician, and it's only going to get worse!

We are barraged these days with negative comments and predictions from doomsayers remarking on the sorry state of healthcare and the need for dramatic reform. Doctors are feeling overburdened and finding it increasingly difficult to practice good medicine. Some physicians are saying they would not go into medicine again and are not recommending it as a career to their children.

I believe that the opposite is true. We now have access to ever-increasing knowledge and tools that enable us to take better care of our patients and improve the health of the general population. Physicians must take advantage of these new capabilities to meet the challenge of practicing medicine in a new environment and adopt a culture of continuous learning and improvement. The changes that are unfolding can allow us to remain true to the values we cherish—diagnosing disease, saving lives, healing the sick, and giving compassionate care—while resulting in much greater impact on our patients and a broader impact on society as a whole.

There is no doubt that over the past two decades a great many changes in the healthcare environment have consumed doctors' time, distracted us from our core task of providing care, and threatened our incomes. More and more criticisms have been leveled at physicians and the healthcare industry. These include concerns about quality, our aging population, the growing number of uninsured, the solvency of Medicare, but mostly, concerns about the runaway costs of medical care.

The nation is focused on the statistics, and we should be too. Currently, the United States has nearly fifty million people without health insurance.[1] Healthcare costs continue to escalate at a rate of about 7 percent per year, more than twice the rate of growth in the overall economy.[2] Projections over the next six to eight years are for similar annual rates of growth, although they have slowed for now because of the 2008 recession.[3] Healthcare constituted 17.9 percent of US GDP in 2010 and is projected to grow to 20 percent by 2020.[4] Total average out-of-pocket spending on healthcare rises steadily while family incomes remain largely unchanged. Employer family premiums equaled 18 percent of the median family income in 2009 and are projected to go to 24 percent by 2020.[5]

It's clear that healthcare costs are on an unsustainable trajectory and that we have to find a way to create greater value with fewer resources. The business community complains that healthcare costs negatively affect their ability to compete in the global market. For example, General Motors now spends more on health premiums (about $1,500 per car) than on steel.[6] The US has the most expensive healthcare system but is ranked near last on quality and other measures when compared to highly industrialized nations. Business productivity is impacted by the poor health status of employees. Baby boomers are starting to retire and enter their most healthcare intensive period, while the working population constitutes a smaller and smaller portion of the population. In fact, in 2012 nearly 20 percent of the US workforce is age fifty-five or older, up from 14 percent in 2002.[7]

Meanwhile, patients' expectations of the healthcare industry and of their physicians are changing. An increasing number of people want more involvement in their own healthcare and want to partner with their physician.

These patients are no longer content to simply accept the physician's diagnosis and treatment plan. They come to their medical appointments armed with a vast amount of information possibly gleaned from the Internet or from the growing number of pharmaceutical advertisements on television. They may want the latest and most expensive treatments, sometimes with little concern about their costs and comparative benefits. And some are willing to take legal action if they don't feel like their needs are met or if something goes wrong.

All these forces make us feel like we're under siege. But I would counsel young people not to give up on medicine as a career choice, or on service as a value. Technological and knowledge advances are making possible a new and more affordable model of high-quality healthcare, and a more satisfying medical practice. Twenty years ago, who would have believed that doctors today operate in a world where they can quickly detect life- or health-threatening changes in a patient's condition through home-based monitoring? Or that a general practitioner in a small town can send images to a specialty center in a big city and call upon a team of doctors to help make sure the patient gets the best diagnosis possible? Or that a physician who has never seen a particular patient before can see her entire medical record before treating her for an emergency condition?

The emerging model will improve quality, increase access to care, control costs, and provide flexibility, while at the same time enhancing the professional lives of physicians. It will promote and enhance wellness, not just care for people when they are sick. Doctors will share information more easily, operate more effectively as a team, and utilize new capabilities for less labor-intensive treatment of illness. We can have the satisfaction of being part of a profession that delivers ever-increasing quality and value to our patients, our families, and our communities. And, we can create more flexibility in our own schedules, allowing the new generation of doctors to achieve a better balance between their work and personal life.

In order to optimize this new model, physicians must overcome their general skepticism and embrace change. What should be our new expectations? This book closely examines the major elements of the newly emerging model of healthcare and the implications for the practice of medicine. There are eight basic elements that are reshaping the practice of medicine. Each places new demands on physicians and offers new opportunities to improve care and enhance professional growth and impact. I give a short description and some examples of each below. By preparing ourselves for these, we can also better contribute to the definition of the ongoing changes in healthcare to fulfill our professional mission and aspirations.

The ideas in this book come from my personal experiences and lessons learned over many years. I was a practicing physician for thirty years in internal medicine, hematology, and oncology. I have held a variety of leadership positions, including serving for eight years as the chief executive officer and chairman of the board for the Southern California Permanente Medical Group (SCPMG). The Southern California Region includes over six thousand physicians and fifty-eight thousand employees caring for almost 3.5 million lives. SCPMG has a long-term relationship and exclusive yearly contract to deliver physician services to members of the Southern California Region of Kaiser Foundation's Health Plan, in conjunction with the Kaiser Foundation Hospitals. I have been fortunate to work with and learn from the remarkable physicians in the Southern California Region of Kaiser Permanente. Together with Kaiser Foundation Hospitals and Health Plan, we have worked to craft a better system for everyone: physicians and other medical care providers, patients, members, and payers.

The KP Promise*

- *Quality you can trust*
- *Caring with a personal touch*
- *Convenient and easy access*
- *Affordability*

Kaiser Permanente Southern California's Values

- *Quality*
- *Service*
- *Results*
- *Integrity*
- *Partnership*
- *Diversity*
- *Accountability*
- *Flexibility*
- *Innovation*

All of Kaiser Permanente has operated under the KP Promise, which is composed of four cornerstones that we strive to incorporate into everything we do.* Kaiser Permanente Southern California has nine values, which we see as critical elements that shape our behavior and our culture, and that we believe lead us to success in what we do. By executing the trends detailed in this book, we fulfill the KP Promise.

During my tenure as CEO, we improved quality and increased access while annually reducing our expense trend. The Southern California Region of Kaiser Permanente (KPSC) now ranks among the top ten nationally in a number of preventive medicine measures (e.g., colorectal cancer screening, breast cancer screening, controlling hypertension, and many others). Providing exceptional preventive medicine saves lives, improves health and reduces costs. To my delight, the

** actively used by some of the KP regions*

public in Southern California has taken note. We enjoyed remarkable growth over the last seven years, increasing our membership every year, even during the nation's worst recession since the 1930s. We've done all that and at the same time have hired more physicians, provided more support to them, and have substantially increased their salaries. See the appendix for some of the overarching achievements we've made in the last seven years.

Some might say that we can't learn from Kaiser Permanente's experiences because it's so unique to KP: it's an integrated system, it's not fee for service, it's an HMO, it's "socialist" medicine, and so on. Some of you might be tempted to close the book now and say, "I'm done with this." But I ask you to give this a second thought. The differences are just the point. The way in which Kaiser Permanente is different has given us an extraordinary opportunity to put in place and learn about new approaches, like evidence-based medicine, integrated care, wellness, prevention, and outcomes-based rewards, which are elements of most reform efforts today. These approaches are needed everywhere. As you'll see throughout the book, we're right in the mainstream of the trends in healthcare. Many healthcare systems are moving in these same directions.

Changing Healthcare—Some of the New Approaches at SCPMG

- *Language program for physicians*
- *Telemedicine*
- *Proactive office encounter*
- *Pay-for-quality-performance incentives*
- *Operating room efficiency program*
- *Mobile health vehicle*
- *Healthy living helpline*
- *Innovation from within*

I believe that the journey my colleagues and I have taken to build a high-value healthcare system is relevant to all physicians. We have had the opportunity for physicians to work with the Hospitals and Health Plans arms of Kaiser Permanente to define changes that enhance the value of the healthcare we provide. Such partnering ensures that physicians can provide high-quality care in a system being crafted by them. Partnering and integration are inherent in the move to accountable care organizations (ACOs) and medical homes that are part of today's healthcare reform initiatives, and we all have to learn to do it right.

We have learned that physicians have to craft and own the systems they work in. In essence, physicians have led the establishment of accountable care in the Southern California region. We have had success with many new, innovative programs that provide more support to our patients and complement the work of physicians. This includes the Proactive Office Encounter (POE), whereby patients who come to any appointment at Kaiser Permanente are reminded of preventive tests or follow-ups that are due, and are immediately given appointments for these (see chapter 2 for a description). Working with our Hospitals and Health Plan colleagues, we have developed a pervasive model of unit-based care. This approach is similar to the medical homes that are being introduced more broadly in US healthcare, which aim to provide comprehensive primary care oriented to the whole person, continuity with a personal physician, enhanced access, and an emphasis on safety and quality.[8] We have implemented a language concordance program that matches non-English-speaking patients with doctors who speak their language and provides language training for interested physicians. SCPMG University is our onboarding program for new doctors. An operating room efficiency program has enabled us to greatly improve access, safety, and quality of surgical procedures. Physicians have led the introduction of these and many other changes.

In introducing change, we have learned what it means to be a physician in the emerging new order—and how to enhance our performance and the outcomes we experience. We have discovered that physicians at all stages of their careers are dedicated to leading change that enables more effective care. Two of our many physician leaders are illustrative of the wide range of perspectives among our doctors, while sharing the common focus on improvement that characterizes the partners of SCPMG:

Dr. Todd Sachs, chief of Surgery at our West Los Angeles Medical Center, has practiced medicine for twenty-six years and has been a leader in implementing significant improvement in our surgical processes.

> *"Change in how we practice medicine has happened fairly recently, but now it's changing rapidly and it will change even more. At Kaiser Permanente we've always focused on preventive care, and we felt we were pretty good. But we didn't have the ability to measure it and to demonstrate that preventive care was the best way to go in terms of outcomes and cost. Once we put metrics in place we found out we were OK, but not great. Now we can also put processes in place to improve prevention. These processes allow us to discover ways to improve how we deliver care in general, and make our members the healthiest possible.*
>
> *Twenty-six years ago I walked in and I just started seeing patients. Now new physicians come in and before they see patients they*

have a three-day course about our electronic medical record. They also attend SCPMG University, where they learn about our values and how we should care for our members. We want to make sure that physicians step up and realize how they play a vital role in proper decision making for the betterment of the care of patients. We were in training for so long—when we come out we need to find our niche within the group and prove our identity. But the most meaningful aspect of being an SCPMG physician is realizing that it is so much more enjoyable to work with *colleagues to take care of our patients and figure out processes to consistently deliver high-quality care."*

Dr. Brian Nguyen has been practicing family medicine for eight years. He quickly became very involved in many of the changes at KPSC, including assuming an additional role as physician director of Clinical Strategic Goals (CSG) at the South Bay Medical Center. He is also a physician representative on our SCPMG Board of Directors and is currently the physician-in-charge of the startup of a large new clinic.

"Younger docs come out of medical school expecting changes. SCPMG's values and outcome orientation have been key. Understanding why we're getting the outcomes we're getting, knowing what the evidence says, and continual improvement are key values. Physicians believe in an outcome orientation and in emulating effective practice. We learn that in medical school. Our system at SCPMG allows us to do this on a much broader scale. I'm very concerned with efficiency. I don't like to see waste in the system. In the past, physicians have held on to the belief that medical knowledge is mysterious and that others can't understand it. We've put a lot of waste in the system through processes that are inefficient and haven't wanted to open the system to scrutiny. We're now getting rid of the steps that don't need to be done—simplifying processes with the help of our EMR and other IT capabilities. Everything is data driven. As a board member I can help identify system-wide issues and work with my colleagues to develop greater clinical capabilities. Younger physicians see this as a challenge. We're willing to adapt and accept the unknown. We're not trying to salvage the old system."

Brian and Todd are physicians in different fields and in different career stages. Yet they both approach the improvement of medicine with remarkable energy, concern, and passion. You'll hear more from them, and from other physician leaders, as you continue through the book.

This book is not about who pays for healthcare. I leave it to the economists and politicians to sort that out. It is about a new model of care that delivers higher value to society, and what this means for the practice of medicine. It is about us—the physicians who are key hubs in the healthcare delivery network—and how we practice.

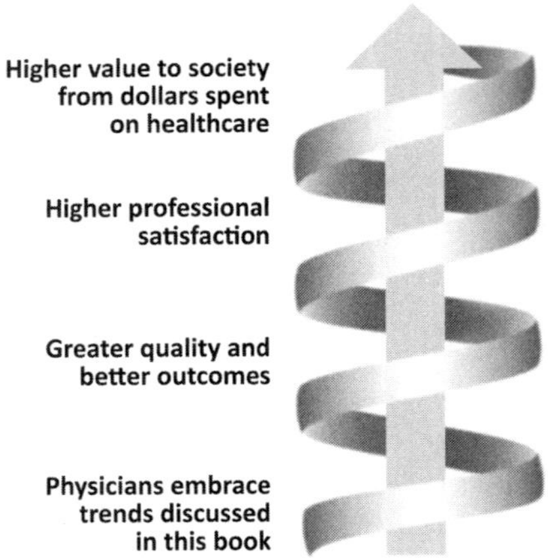

Figure 1:
A virtuous cycle from embracing the trends in this book

This book is not about who pays for healthcare. I leave it to the economists and politicians to sort that out. It is about a new model of care that delivers higher value to society, and what this means for the practice of medicine. It is about us—the physicians who are key hubs in the healthcare delivery network—and how we practice. In my view, we physicians can and must make sure that the trends I talk about in this book add up to significantly greater quality, better outcomes, and higher value to society from the dollars spent on healthcare—and to higher professional satisfaction. This is true no matter the setting we practice in—whether in private practice, as members of physician groups, in HMOs, large or small healthcare systems, community hospitals and clinics, the Veterans Administration system, specialty facilities, accountable healthcare collectives, or company-managed clinics.

Quality and Value: Keys to a Sustainable Healthcare System

All around the world, the issues of healthcare quality and value are being debated in a context of growing need and proportionately shrinking resources.[9] Don Berwick, the former administrator of the Centers for Medicare and Medicaid Services and president and chief executive of the Institute for Healthcare Improvement, has written and worked tirelessly to get healthcare systems to be able to achieve what he calls the "Triple Aim": improving the care experience, improving our population's health, and reducing the cost of healthcare.[10] As the American healthcare reform bill (the Patient Protection and Affordable Care Act, often shortened to ACA) is implemented, the simultaneous demand for quality and value are increasingly central to the debates. The bill has already stimulated widespread experimentation with accountable care organizations (ACOs) to provide measurably higher quality care at lower cost. (An ACO is a network of doctors and hospitals that share responsibility for providing comprehensive care to a defined population of patients and are incentivized to deliver quality healthcare while keeping costs down.)[11] Health plans and other payers are starting to offer incentives to hospitals and physicians to meet quality standards and to continually improve the value they deliver. Pennsylvania's Geisinger Health System's pay for performance program, for example, offers incentives for caregivers to follow established best practices that have been shown to relate to outcomes.[12] Martin's Point Healthcare, a physician-led primary healthcare system in New England, is successfully using incentives for targeted purposes such as to spur on its primary care physicians to deliver improved diabetes care.[13] The Integrated Healthcare Association's P4P initiatives have included the development of standardized metrics that serve as the basis of the performance-based pay of a number of healthcare plans in Los Angeles, including the HealthCare

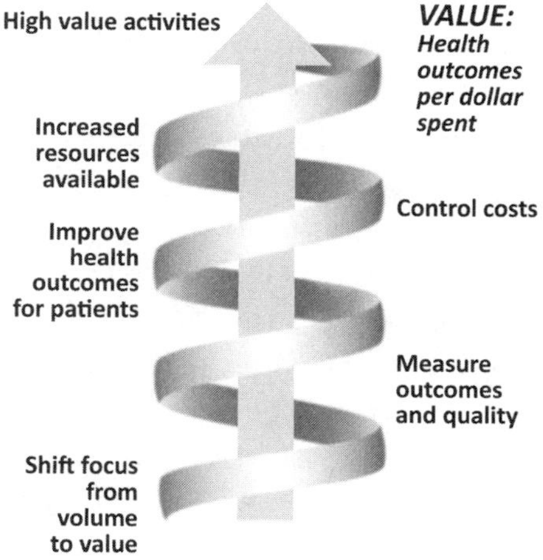

Figure 2:
The shift to value

Partners medical group.† We are all getting used to quality measure reporting programs and groups such as Healthcare Effectiveness Data and Information Set (HEDIS), the Five-Star Quality Rating System for Medicare Advantage Plans, the Consumer Assessment of Healthcare Providers and Systems (CAHPS), and the Integrated Healthcare Association (IHA).

Against the opposition of many physicians, the healthcare reform bill debate also began to explore the shift to value as the basis for reimbursement—departing from the longstanding habits of fees for volume and services.[14] The goal is to achieve high value for patients and society—using limited healthcare dollars to more effectively increase health status and quality of life. Doctors will be paid based on value, not volume—perhaps at first mostly for Medicare beneficiaries. But the genie is out of the bottle. For example, Geisinger Health System has a bundled payment system that incentivizes outcomes, not activity levels. The explicit goal is to increase value: to achieve increased outcomes and quality of care for patients for the same or lower costs.[15] Indeed, the state of Massachusetts is working on legislation to replace the fee-for-service system with a system of flat global payments that would incent physicians to keep patients well.[16] The concept of bundling payments instead of the standard fee-for-service is here to stay.[17] We all have to make sure we are part of an effective system and work with each other more efficiently and collaboratively.

What this means is unknown for most of us, scary for some, and anathema for others. No matter what our political beliefs and ideologies, and no matter what funding approaches unfold through time, it is clear that society expects increases in quality and value. I believe the move to value also lines up with what physicians want—no one wants to practice bad medicine! Nobody wants a bad outcome. We go to medical school to learn to help patients become or stay healthy. We now have the tools and knowledge to achieve both quality and value—and this affords great opportunity and creates great challenges for us all.

In order to optimize value, we must overcome our general skepticism and embrace these changes. This book will closely examine the major elements of the newly emerging model of healthcare and the implications for practicing physicians. If you're just starting out your medical practice, these are the trends that are shaping the environment in which you will practice. If you're an established physician, these are the trends that have been changing

† See http://www.iha.org for more information.

much that you had come to expect about the way medicine is practiced.

Each of the eight elements that are reshaping healthcare places new demands on physicians but offers new opportunities to improve care and enhance professional growth.

1. Prevention and Wellness

Why do we wait until someone becomes sick to interact with him or her? Why don't we set out from the very start to promulgate the idea of health throughout society? Why don't we look at the whole person and work to make that person's whole life an experience of health and well-being?

We are well aware of the power of prevention in promoting health, improving quality of life, and reducing the overwhelming demand on our healthcare resources. We also know that there are great challenges in achieving healthier lifestyles, earlier detection of disease, and better life-cycle care conducive to health and well-being. People around the world are living longer and becoming heavier and less physically active. The median age of the population of almost every country in the world is increasing.[18] Our healthcare system is coping with more and more chronic conditions that drain its (and our) time, energy, and resources. Two-thirds of all Americans are either overweight or obese.[19] The World Health Organization notes that "worldwide obesity has more than doubled since 1980"—in 2008, over 1.4 billion adults, age twenty and older, were overweight.[20] Kids and adults are also much more physically inactive, at school, at work, and at home, and "low levels of physical fitness are associated with markedly increased... mortality rates."[21] We're practicing medicine in a new era–an era where we can only make headway by influencing our patients to take responsibility for their own health.

The sad reality is that the US medical care system is overpriced and ineffective because it is designed to wait for people to become sick before they are treated. There is some indication that this is beginning to change. Hospital admissions of Medicare patients with heart failure fell by 30 percent between 1999 and 2008, and there has been a 23 percent decline in Medicare admissions for heart attacks. Obesity rates have stabilized and smoking rates have declined.[22] Yet the statistics are still far too high, and lifestyle issues are impacting the health of our population beginning at very young ages.

We have to become champions of wellness and prevention. We can't control the cost of healthcare or deliver high-value care without putting wellness and prevention front and center. Wellness is the "real deal." As a society and a profession we badly need to prevent illness where we can and prevent rapid escalation of severity where we can't. We need to align the incentives in the system toward health, not illness. This will enable physicians to use our extensive expertise where it is most needed. Of course many people will nonetheless move along the chronic disease continuum, but hopefully more slowly and with fewer flare-ups and more infrequent need for repetitive medical intervention. We'll have the satisfaction of being part of a system that promotes wellness and quality of life. Obviously physicians can't do this alone, but we can take leadership roles in a system oriented to health.

The concept of wellness is beginning to take root in society, in some measure because improving health status is an economic imperative. Productivity at work is impacted not just by absenteeism, but also by time lost to presentee-ism (going to work while sick and consequently not being productive).[23] Healthy employees and citizens are the lifeblood of our societal and economic wherewithal—and it is they, and not the sick and injured, who are the source of the resources that pay for our healthcare systems and our livelihoods. Deteriorating health status can greatly impact our economic competitiveness and can bring our health systems to their knees. We could easily get into a cycle of decreasing resources significantly caused by our failure to promote a healthy population. The lives of physicians would then get worse, not better.

These prognoses are leading to changes in employer health benefit plans to emphasize wellness.[24] The stark economic consequences of our current system are the burning platform behind the debates associated with the US healthcare reform legislation. Prevention and wellness cover the whole continuum of care—and can't be addressed in a fragmented system where no one is attending to overall health status. We physicians can no longer say "that's not our job." Chapter two will explore what this means for us.

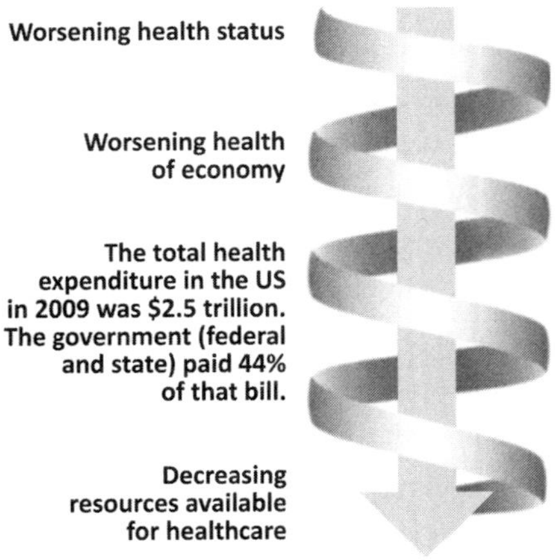

Figure 3:
The death spiral of bad health and increasing cost (Data source: National Health Expenditures 2009 Highlights, http://www.cms.gov/NationalHealthExpendData/downloads/highlights.pdf)

2. Patient-Centered Care

To the layperson, it must seem absurd that physicians are only now starting to locate patients in the center of their focus. What in the world were we looking at before? Just as healthcare is expanding its focus from disease to include wellness, we doctors are also simultaneously widening our focus from the disease itself to the person standing in front of us. In doing so, we can better comprehend the patient's perspective. Medical schools have even started to teach students how to improve communication and listening skills in order to develop a good bedside manner.[25] When I attended medical school, it was left to chance.

Medicine is a service-oriented profession, and it's getting more competitive. The online resource Angie's List ranks plumbers, landscapers, limo services—and doctors.[‡] In general, patients are expecting more than they used to, and they no longer have unquestioning respect for our judgment or motives. We have to *earn* their respect.

Somewhat reluctantly, we have begun to share power and responsibility with patients, who become proactive partners in addressing their own health challenges.[26] I believe this partnership will make our job both easier and more rewarding. Patient-centered care is a powerful and necessary development that should result not only in improving the doctor-patient relationship, but in improving quality outcomes.[27]

We bemoan the fact that it sometimes seems like patients come to a consultation just to tell doctors what to do. In reality, because of widespread pharmaceutical advertising and the proliferation of medical information on the web, patients do have the ability to become quite well-informed about their conditions even before they set foot in our examining rooms.[28] Is that really a bad thing? Moving to a patient-centered approach dovetails with the drive for wellness very well. Wellness looks at the whole person; it requires the individual to be proactive in monitoring and nurturing his or her own health and to be knowledgeable about how to do so. We need to take advantage of our patients' eagerness to learn about their own condition and to be involved in decisions about how that care will proceed. I will talk more about patient-centered care in chapter three.

3. Electronic Medical Records and Other IT Applications

It has become widely understood that access to complete medical records is integral to high-quality healthcare. The American Recovery and Reinvestment

‡ See http://www.angieslist.com/services.aspx for the complete list of physician, dentist, and other healthcare specialties that can be reviewed on the site.

Act (ARRA) of 2009 (through the Health Information Technology for Economic and Clinical Health (HITECH) provisions of the bill) will penalize any US healthcare provider who hasn't started using electronic medical records (EMRs) by 2015 through a reduction in their Medicaid and Medicare payments.[29] Many integrated systems, including Kaiser Permanente, the Mayo Clinic, Cleveland Clinic, Geisinger, and the Veterans Administration, have a leg up on creating integrated EMRs, but we are also seeing rapidly increasing adoption in the community-based fee-for-service arena. The increasing efforts to achieve interoperability between systems are a testimony to the importance of EMRs to high-quality care. One example is the Care Connectivity Consortium (Geisinger Health System, Kaiser Permanente, Mayo Clinic, Intermountain Healthcare, and Group Health Cooperative) that has developed and begun to implement safe and secure ways to share data across their disparate EMRs.[30]

For our medical group, EMR implementation was frustrating and demanding as we all had to change habits, enter data into the system, and accept that our patients' records are available not only to us, but to others who care for them so that they can get the most knowledgeable care no matter where in the region they are being treated. (Of course, we do still have some privacy walls in place electronically, such as for psychiatric records). We're exposed, and this data transparency can seem threatening. Yet we now agree that these records provide each of us the opportunity to know more about our patients and their history, and to make better medical decisions. They provide a basis for coordination and integration of care. They allow us to work better with each other, and to deliver better care.

New information technologies have also made it possible for us to break the syndrome of patients needing office visits to detect the need for and initiate routine assessments. Virtual tracking, monitoring, and screening patients to detect needed intervention are becoming more common. Patients have the option to receive most of their test results electronically and automatically. Our mix of face-to-face, voice-to-voice and electronic work and patient interface is changing, and we are developing new expectations of what it means to practice medicine. Chapter four will take a further look at information and transparency.

4. Goals, Measurements and Accountability

Tracking outcomes on all levels—hospitals, clinics, specialties, medical groups, and on down to individual physicians—is now quite possible, and society is now requiring that we do so. This enables patients, insurers, the government and others to better measure value. We've learned at SCPMG that measuring quality and outcomes and continually improving healthcare processes helps us deliver greater value to society. And, it increases the pride we all feel in the care we deliver. Using our EMR and other information systems, we've been able to set goals and track metrics that have allowed us to demonstrate continual improvement in the outcomes for our patients and other stakeholders. We have been able to focus our whole system on improving these outcomes. Together, we have made changes in the way we practice that have moved our system to be ranked in the top ten by HEDIS in controlling high blood pressure, cervical cancer screening, cholesterol management, and comprehensive diabetes care, among others.

These measurement systems bring unprecedented transparency and visibility to physicians' work, and put more pressure and more accountability on doctors than ever before. Yet they also enable the rewarding of quality and outcomes and linking physician compensation to improvements and performance. This is something that is mandated by the US healthcare reform bill, becoming effective in 2015.[31] More importantly, it lines up the incentives in the system with quality and the value that our profession delivers. Chapter five will look further at the impact of metrics and accountability on the practice of healthcare.

5. Keeping Up to Date: Evidence-Based Practice and Continuing Medical Education

Human brains do not evolve as quickly as medical knowledge and technology do. Our internal mental hardware works as it has for fifty thousand years or so. A physician or healthcare provider may want to keep abreast of the latest medical discoveries, breakthroughs, and controversies, but it is becoming impossible for individuals to be perfectly well informed about everything in their area of practice. As the Institute of Medicine notes in its influential brief, *Crossing the Quality Chasm*, there is "more to know, more to do, more to manage, more to watch, and more people involved" in healthcare now.[32] It's not surprising that advances in this gigantic, complex system are often not noted and adopted into practice by healthcare practitioners. Wildly inconsistent treatment by region has been documented in the US by the Dartmouth Atlas of Healthcare.[§] We doctors are incredibly busy, and

§ *Online at http://www.dartmouthatlas.org/*

it may seem easier just to treat a condition the way we were trained. All of this is easy to understand but distressing and hard to stomach. What this means for patients is that they may not be receiving the best care for any given condition, even while incurring rapidly escalating costs.

Evidence-based practice has come into the mainstream of medical practice over the last couple of decades to help with this problem of assimilating and using best practices. While never a substitute for physician judgment, guidelines for best practices can bypass the shortcomings of individual human memory and help us become better aware of the overwhelming amount of information available to physicians. Yet such guidelines will always lag behind current knowledge and changing capabilities, and physicians become comfortable with their way of practicing medicine and have limited time to individually explore new guidelines. As knowledge generation accelerates, we all need to be part of rich communities of practice that share knowledge and explore the evidence about what really is effective. Our careers span generations of medical advances. Part of the professionalism of being a physician is continuous learning. We all need strategies for accessing and incorporating new knowledge and that includes shared learning, learning without walls, and studying to get board recertified. Chapter six will talk about how new standards of accountability combined with ever-escalating knowledge are changing medical practice.

6. Innovation and Improvement

Innovation is a critical element in any industry. The field of medicine has advanced through great innovations in diagnostic and treatment approaches, made possible by ever-increasing knowledge about the human body and its systems and the burgeoning fields of diagnostic and therapeutic electronics that enable interventions unheard of just decades ago. Yet the fundamental organization of healthcare has only recently begun to change to reflect the new realities relating to increased demand and the availability of ever-increasing modes of treatment.

The pressures on medical systems will only increase, and sustaining high-quality healthcare will be the responsibility of everyone. We physicians can no longer expect everyone else to change around us. Healthcare needs continuing innovation to ensure that we are not only organized to use the skills and resources of our healthcare system to best meet the needs of our patients, but that we can continually generate new knowledge and develop increasingly effective treatments. Given physicians' roles in the healthcare system, our knowledge and perspectives are critical to successful innovation.

Not all of us will be innovators, but knowledge and capabilities are growing so quickly that healthcare systems need physicians who innovate and blaze the path for others. Refining and implementing new approaches is an opportunity and responsibility for all physicians. Chapter seven will explore what it means for the practice of medicine that the healthcare system will be continuously changing and innovating. Some of this will be quite disruptive.

7. Integration and Teamwork

Physicians don't work in isolation. We are hubs in complex networks of care deliverers and are only as effective as the teams we build and the relationships we maintain. Halvorson and Isham describe the current landscape as "millions of independent, uncoordinated, separately motivated moving parts, each with its own economic priorities and self-focused financial goals."[33] They aren't exaggerating. Different departments in the same hospital, an external medical office, and a dentist may all see the same person for problems that may well be intimately linked and yet never talk to each other or see medical records other than their own. When a patient has a chronic condition that encompasses more than one health issue, interconnected care only makes sense to treat the totality of the problem, yet this type of illness often doesn't get treated holistically.[34]

To use our time and society's healthcare dollars wisely, we need to coordinate better to avoid the problems of poor quality and redundancy. The EMR makes it possible for physicians to operate as part of an extended team that can draw on each other's knowledge. Patients can receive appropriate care from providers knowledgeable about them as individuals, and about the treatment they are receiving from others. We can better use the skills and knowledge of our team members to do many of the routine tasks that overwhelm physicians but don't call upon their deep expertise. This can free us up for the more uncertain and judgmental decisions and expertise-based processes that we are trained to do. Teams enable doctors, so we can deliver the value that society expects from us. Chapter eight will examine the kinds of teams and networks in which physicians are increasingly working, and the impact on their practice.

8. Leadership

Doctors must step up and lead. We actually do this every day, whether we think about it or not. As soon as we put on a white coat, we are leaders. Effective physicians are day-to-day leaders in the teams in which they work. How we relate to the others upon whom we and our patients depend is a major factor in the quality of care and the value that we provide. Leadership involves modeling what is important, communicating clear expectations, sharing information and building our team, and appreciating the knowledge, perspectives, and contributions of the people who work with and support us. Other members of the healthcare team also rely on us to lead—just as we rely on them to manage their part of the complex process of delivering high-quality care. This leadership role is the key ingredient of high-performing healthcare systems.

The patients under our care depend on our experience and knowledge, but they also rely on us to lead them and our team. Too often we treat the presenting symptoms and disease states without providing leadership to the patient and the family who need to be encouraged to make changes in their lives in order to recuperate, prevent illness, or enhance their quality of life. We avoid the hard discussions. We don't take the time to make sure patients are connected to other team members and resources. We leave that to the patient who must navigate between disconnected and often disaffected providers. Systems such as Palmetto Health Hospitals in South Carolina,[35] Presbyterian Healthcare Services in New Mexico, and many cancer centers are using nurse navigators, who help cancer patients through the medical system and provide information, advice, and support.[36] While such roles are important, we physicians cannot expect them to substitute for our leadership role in making sure the entire healthcare team is oriented to these same tasks.

We also have to be willing to be led. Physicians are professionals, and we don't like to be told what to do by administrators and managers. We come out of medical school thinking we know everything! In actuality we have very deep knowledge that enables us to achieve outcomes that were inconceivable only decades ago—and yet in many cases to be humbled by illness and deterioration of the human body in the face of which we are powerless. We are dependent on contributions from many others, who can help patients work through some of the complicating factors that may be associated with their disease that can have significant impact on their overall health status and the efficacy of our treatment. Pain, depression, drug dependence, nutritional deficiencies, fear, unemployment, poverty, and confusion are but a few of these areas that our particular specialty knowledge may not address. The improvement of our capabilities to make a difference in the lives of our patients requires coordinated activity among many, and ongoing change in how we work together to address the whole person.

Physicians have a lot of complaints about administrators' decisions that we feel make it more difficult for us to do our jobs. This will only change if physician leaders step up to the plate and co-plan the changes that are occurring in healthcare systems. At SCPMG, we decided that we physicians needed to be leaders in driving change and working with administrators and the Health Plans arm of Kaiser Permanente to define approaches that work. Like HealthCare Partners and many other systems, our physician leaders at every level are teamed with managerial leaders to continually improve the system and focus on outcomes and value. As the societal trends demand more effective and efficient approaches to prevention and treatment, physicians must share the leadership required to make sure they work in high performing systems that continually improve their capabilities. It is no longer possible to say, "We're fine; let others figure out how to pay for our services and deal with the problems of healthcare." This effectively disempowers *us*, the central players in delivering high-quality healthcare.

Being able to share leadership with administrators, other physicians, and other providers is critical in the rapidly changing environment for healthcare. Societal resource trends are clear. Change *will and must* happen, no matter what political party is in power. If physicians don't lead and aren't led by each other, other stakeholders will gladly assume the leadership role and change in healthcare will be thrust upon us. Chapter nine explores what this means for the practice of medicine.

The Plan for This Book

In the chapters that follow, I will develop each of the eight elements of the emerging role of physicians, providing more context and examples from my own and other's experiences. These changes are driven by the undeniable need to increase quality and the value provided by our healthcare systems in order for the system to be sustainable. Prevention and wellness, patient-focused care, emphasis on value and outcomes—who can argue that increasing these would greatly enhance the contribution of our profession to society? Transparency of data, enhanced coordination and teamwork, evidence-based practice, and innovation to improve outcomes and value—the logic of these approaches and their efficacy in improving system performance has been discovered in all work systems. However, they have only recently begun to be applied to healthcare work systems.

We are central contributors in a sector of the economy that enables all other sectors to operate effectively and that impacts the quality of life and health status of all members of the society. This is a heavy responsibility. We often feel buffeted by change, but seldom have or take the time to reflect on why this is happening. I believe we owe it to ourselves and our patients to think about what we can do to make these changes work in our interests and the interests of providing great healthcare. This book is intended to catalyze this reflection—and to give us all a chance to think about our roles and practices in the context of the inevitable change that is affecting us all. The amount of flux in the system provides us with an unprecedented opportunity to make a difference. Everyone can win.

Medicine is the noblest of professions. As you read these pages, I hope you find something that raises your spirits and rekindles your joy. In writing this book, I enjoyed reflecting on my many years as a practicing doctor and physician leader. Our journey at KPSC has had many twists and turns, but in the end is producing extraordinary results. I believe the trusted physician axiom of "do no harm" must be transformed into "do great benefit."

It's an exciting time to be a physician!

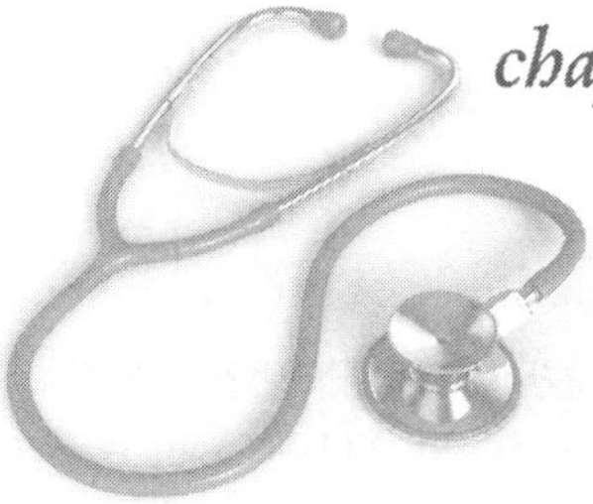

chapter two

Prevention and Wellness

The alarm clock rings, and you can't believe it's that time again—time to get up and get going. We all have a morning routine. And a lot of us bargain with ourselves, "Just thirty minutes more, and then I'll get out of bed." What if instead we jumped up, put on our workout gear and went out for a morning walk or run, or hopped on a stationary bike? Thirty minutes later our endorphins would be flowing and our bodies humming. We would be really ready to start a new day. Sounds great to me! I certainly want this for my patients, my family, coworkers, and myself.

These aren't the ramblings of an idealist, but rather the philosophy that we as physicians should embrace if we are to fulfill the promise of modern medical care to society. We all have different roles in the healthcare system, but all of us can focus on prevention and wellness. Some of us deal with the primary care needs of patients to monitor their overall health status and preventive measures. Some attend to the routine outbreaks of treatable illness and flare-ups of chronic illness, and some identify conditions that need more specialized treatment. We're the first line of defense against unnecessary illness and inappropriate treatment. Some of us have deep specialty knowledge and treat the sickest and most vulnerable of the population and provide advanced interventions to those who have experienced traumatic illness and injury. We try to restore health and functioning, prevent recurrence, and slow progression.

We all entered the profession with the intent of helping people be as healthy as possible and experience the highest quality of life. Yet we've managed as a society and as a profession to create a healthcare system that focuses on sickness, not wellness. I believe that this is changing and that's a major reason why I think this is a great time to be a physician.

Moving Away From the Sickness Model of Healthcare

Nowadays doctors are mainly incentivized to think about something completely different than the overarching view of a person in the best health possible. Doctors practicing medicine routinely only focus on the symptom or the illness we encounter in the examining room, such as the patient who presents with a swollen knee, or a lung mass detected on an x-ray. The patient has become only a host for the illnesses and disease we treat. That just isn't right. It's narrow, shortsighted and it isn't in the best interests of the patient. It uses resources poorly because care is fragmented.

Medical systems focus almost exclusively on diagnosing and treating disease and injury. In the traditional model of healthcare delivery, doctors and other healthcare workers are most likely to connect with patients when they are ill. Indeed, we have learned how to accomplish great medical feats. The application of increasingly sophisticated drugs and technologies, such as robots, lasers, biologics, and ever more sophisticated imaging technologies, has resulted in our ability to save and prolong lives, restore health, and repair bodies in ways inconceivable decades ago. Don't get me wrong, I would never advocate turning our backs on the medicines, techniques and technologies that have been developed over the years. In fact, it is clearly our obligation to make the most efficacious treatment available to our patients and society as a whole. But we are also obligated to build a medical care system that is focused on prevention and wellness.

We physicians need to lead the way in a system that engages people before they get sick, treats them before they get sicker, and focuses on health and well-being as the primary outcomes. Doing so will reduce risk factors, prevent disease, lower healthcare costs, make insurance more affordable, and save lives. By reducing unnecessary illness and treatment, our skills and knowledge will have greater impact on the populations we serve. In some cases we'll be able to treat patients when they are in earlier stages of disease, and thus healthier, and our treatments will be more efficacious. We will experience the satisfaction of achieving the aspirations we had when we entered medical school to relieve illness and suffering, and to save lives. Prevention is not flashy or exciting, and does not grab headlines, but it is big! I believe it is the answer to the American healthcare system's rising costs that are failing to result in world-leading quality.

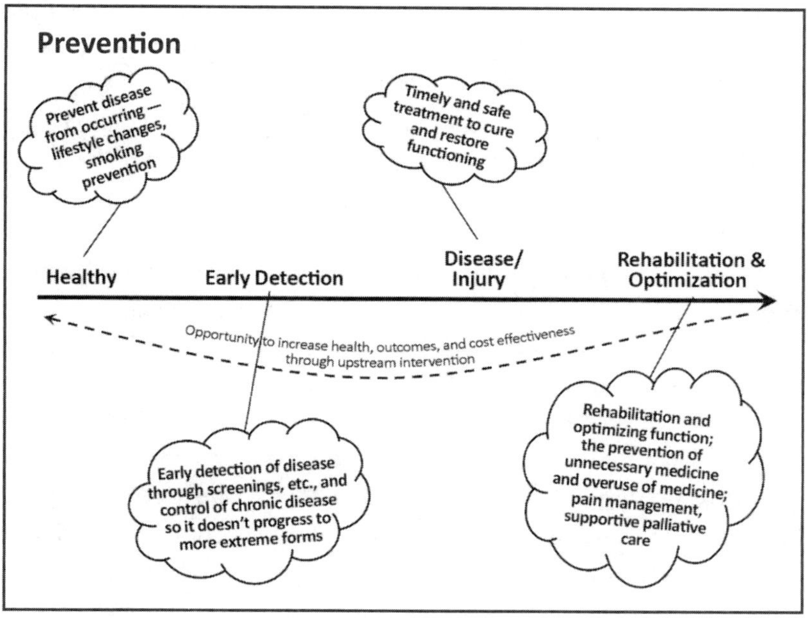

Figure 1: *Timeline of Health*

Moving "upstream" in the disease process has a huge potential return on investment, yet in the US, people are receiving only half of the preventive care that they should be getting.[1] It's been estimated that only 5 percent of the money spent annually on healthcare goes toward preventing disease and promoting wellness.[2] This is starting to change. Prevention is a major priority of the ACA and will receive funding from several of its initiatives.[3] The ACA will also lead to a health promotion/prevention strategy for the entire country. Those who are trying to figure out how our healthcare dollars can deliver greater value—the government, employers, insurers, and enlightened consumers—are beginning to understand the close connection between prevention, health, and cost.

I personally became strongly focused on creating a prevention-oriented system eight years ago after reading Jim Collins' book, *Good to Great*. It is based on the premise that all great organizations figure out what they can be best at. When I became the executive medical director of SCPMG, I found a team of very talented physicians eager to work with me to build a system that excels in prevention in order to greatly increase the health and well-being of the population we serve.

We quickly discovered the magnitude of the challenge. Attending a meeting of physician leaders, I found it disheartening to realize that the Southern California region had low breast cancer screening rates compared to other KP regions. The medical establishment has known for decades that this screening can save lives, reduce suffering, and save money. One in eight women in the US will face a diagnosis of breast cancer; and it is an issue that every woman thinks about. And yet we were not fully vigilant about early detection and prevention.

We embarked on an intensive screening program for breast cancer to put the focus on this number one issue facing women. Our screening rate is now almost 90 percent. Our five year survival rate for breast cancer is 89 percent and we estimate that we save 185 lives per year through our aggressive screening practices. Thankfully, we have advanced state of the art treatments —adjuvant chemotherapy, radiotherapy, breast conservation surgery, and reconstructive surgery—for patients in need. But are we not better off as a healthcare system and as a society to prevent advanced disease and minimize the exposure to treatment modalities that involve significant physical and emotional trauma and life disruption, and sometimes result in long-lasting side effects?

Seeing the power of prevention, physicians throughout the organization began to focus on achieving leadership in other important preventive care areas. Each subspecialty area identified an area to become a leader within the American healthcare system. Orthopedic surgery developed the Healthy Bones Program, an osteoporosis program to prevent bone fractures for all members, and especially for people at risk. Twenty-five percent of women over age sixty-five with hip or femur fractures die, and 20 percent never regain full physical capacity. Healthy Bones prevented over one thousand hip fractures and saved over 250 lives in 2008 alone. Millions of dollars are being saved. We are now number one in the nation in the management and treatment of osteoporosis. This was another win for our patients and physicians!

In my years of caring for hematology oncology patients, I certainly treated my share of patients with advanced colorectal cancer. Even though we have the ability to treat these patients with the most advanced chemotherapeutic regimens, except in the rarest of situations, they finally lost their battles and their lives. I envisioned setting up a screening program where we could eliminate advanced colorectal cancer. Our system in KPSC spends over $150 million yearly in chemotherapy for the treatment of this malignancy. It certainly would be better for all to invest in prevention and allow patients to forego the morbidity associated with chemotherapeutic treatment of an advanced cancer. Our aggressive outreach program uses immunochemical fecal occult blood tests, a more expensive but also a more effective test than standard fecal occult testing, and easier and more convenient for patients. Our screening rates have grown from 52.5 percent to over 70 percent, and stage IV colon cancer has decreased by 31 percent (see figure 2). In our system alone, this equates to saving 4,724 lives per decade. This is yet another success story for patients and care providers. We are treating more patients and getting to them earlier in the cycle—and thus are able to cure more of them.

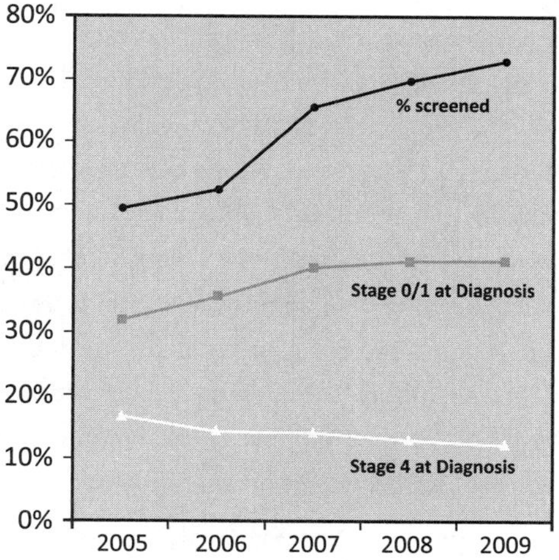

Figure 2: *Impact of Preventive Screening:*
Annual Colorectal Cancer Screening Results Among Fifty- to Eighty-Year-Old SCPMG Members

These are examples where we redirected resources and attention upstream in the disease cycle in order to reduce the incidence of hugely expensive downstream care—care that consumes inordinate amounts of healthcare resources and that is associated with significant loss of productivity, lower quality of life, and lower than optimal outcomes. I do not for one moment believe that such prevention will eliminate the need for the extraordinary capabilities that characterize modern healthcare. The burgeoning population of baby boomers is reaching the age where many more will develop colorectal and other cancers, as well as other debilitating diseases. We need to make sure that we detect these diseases as early as possible and that we prevent unnecessary suffering. This will allow us to wisely use our most sophisticated techniques and the hours of our most advanced specialists for maximum impact on the well-being of our population. This will be a significant accomplishment for our profession.

Preventive Prescriptions

We all need to contribute to prevention. It's a mindset and set of behaviors that needs to permeate the full spectrum of care. Prevention is not the sole purview of specialized roles such as health educators and helpline nurses, although they play an important role as members of the healthcare team. We should all seek to practice where these resources are available to support our patients and our own efforts. In addition, prevention is not the focus only of primary care physicians, while specialists worry only about treating acutely ill patients or people with complex medical issues. It's all of our responsibility. We physicians can have tremendous influence by focusing patients and the whole healthcare team on prevention.

Healthcare providers need to excel in four areas of prevention: instilling healthy lifestyles, preventing or minimizing the impact of acute illness, slowing chronic disease progression, and reducing or eliminating adverse outcomes in the hospital. I coined the phrase "Preventive Prescriptions" and am fond of referring to the figure below that reminds us that we physicians can prescribe more than treatment—we can prescribe preventive measures in these four areas.

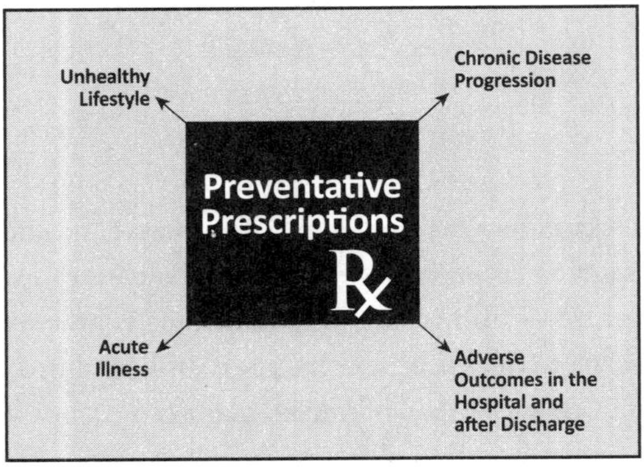

Figure 3: *Preventive Prescriptions*

Healthy Lifestyle

First and foremost is healthy living, encompassing such things as smoking cessation, reducing excessive alcohol intake, and paying attention to nutrition and exercise. Healthy living is an important prescription for our members no matter what their current health status is and no matter the purpose for which we are seeing them. For example, we as physicians understand the ravages of smoking and its consequences for both the healthy and the acutely ill. Nineteen percent of Americans smoke, and second-hand smoke affects us all. Similarly, alcohol is more and more prevalent in American culture and is adversely permeating our schools and colleges.

The obesity epidemic has no end in sight. The two-thirds of all Americans who are overweight or obese often have coexisting conditions such as hypertension, glucose intolerance, and sleep apnea.[4] Obesity is associated with an increased risk of death from cardiovascular disease, diabetes, kidney disease, and some forms of cancer.[5] Sadly, it's not just adults we have to worry about. Kids are also heavier and much more physically inactive, at school, at work, and at home. Because of their excess weight, "growing numbers of children now have diseases once considered to be 'adult' conditions, such as type 2 diabetes, nonalcoholic fatty liver disease, and hypertension."[6]

We physicians should not see these trends as beyond our influence. We should not accept the inevitability that we treat people after they have become obese and inactive and have started the cycle of chronic disease. Certainly, bariatric surgery is no panacea. The procedure carries significant risks, and it doesn't address why people get obese: their lifestyle choices. The real answer in most cases comes down to weight management, exercise, and nutrition. We all know what vital signs to measure at a patient's appointment: pulse, BP, temperature, weight—and to that we at SCPMG have added exercise. We proactively ask our patients if they exercise thirty minutes five days a week. In addition, we can refer patients to our Healthy Living Helpline. The wellness coaches on the Helpline are a multidisciplinary team of nurses, registered dietitians, licensed social workers and health educators. The Helpline encounter is downloaded into our EMR so all providers are aware of, and can reinforce, the care plan.

We have successfully piloted using health educators as team members in pediatric departments to proactively engage kids and parents in waiting rooms. These roles are intended to reinforce efforts by physicians to stimulate healthier lifestyles. Health educators provide information and sign people up for the Healthy Family Club, which focuses on exercise and nutrition. Our goal is to prevent a whole host of problems, in the short term and later in life, and to help our members to live happier and healthier lives.

Fundamentally, healthy living is the responsibility of patients and families. Yet we physicians can be a much more potent force for healthy eating and physical activity. We cannot do this alone. Ideally we are part of a team of providers that gives due attention to these issues. We have great opportunity to significantly improve people's health and save money at the same time when we focus on prevention in a systematic way, both in preventing the diseases from actually occurring at all, and in how we manage disease if it has already manifested.

Preventing Acute Disease

The second preventive prescription is to prevent acute disease, or to detect it early enough to lessen its severity and impact. This could be through screening tests to detect early breast or colon cancer, or for chlamydia. It could be via a vaccination for preventing herpes zoster or pneumonia. It could be vigilance about overutilization of drugs with life-threatening side effects or detecting when drugs are interfering with each other. Or it could be through regular check-ups and easier access to medical care. For example, in Michigan, Priority Health and a coalition of community stakeholders have found ways to make routine and preventive care accessible to children on Medicaid through an initiative called the Children's Healthcare Access Program. It creates medical homes for these children and has significantly increased the number of same-day visits. This has reduced pediatric inpatient hospital use by 17 percent, reduced emergency room visits by 6.2 percent, and measurably improved such health outcomes as asthma control.[7]

At KPSC we quickly realized that all outreach efforts on prevention cannot be placed on the shoulders of primary care physicians. In fact, after we analyzed the nature of our patient visits, we were somewhat surprised to see that two-thirds were visits to see specialists, not primary care physicians. Despite our initial assumption that primary care physicians and their teams should be responsible for ensuring that patients get preventive care, the majority of our opportunities to personally connect with patients are with specialists. It is *all* of our responsibility to be vigilant about needed preventive measures.

We wanted our entire healthcare system to focus on prevention, and to reach out to provide maximum support to patients to make sure it happens. We realized that we could lighten the load on physicians by involving the entire care team in the prevention process. Our Proactive Office Encounter (POE) gets our whole system focused on prevention—even those in clinical settings that see the sickest of patients and provide the most specialized of care. Care providers routinely and proactively pull up our patients' electronic medical records at every visit, discuss with them what prevention initiatives or care gaps need to be addressed, and immediately schedule the appointments. This occurs at every visit in every department. By involving our entire care team, caregivers other than just physicians have the satisfaction of becoming engaged in wellness and prevention.

Worldwide, annual influenza epidemics hit an estimated three to five million people, and kill between two hundred fifty thousand and five hundred thousand.[8] In the United States, estimates range between three thousand and forty-nine thousand deaths per year.[9] To prevent or mitigate this potentially devastating disease, KPSC uses a combination of strategies to get our members immunized, notably special outreach efforts to parents of babies under two and preteens—and the powerful vehicle of the POE. We ask all of our physicians to get a flu shot, and to become active advocates of this with their patients. We have also worked to increase our rate of childhood immunizations. Our Combo 3 immunization rate improved 5.24 percent from 2009 to 2011, and now stands at 85.1 percent. This improvement means 1,348 more children have received their immunizations.

I believe that all physicians want to be part of a system that is focused on prevention and one that provides support and shares responsibility for this. Such a work system enables us to feel confident that our patients' preventive

Prevention: Two Physicians' Views

Dr. Todd Sachs, Chief of Surgery for West Los Angeles

"We get used to our worlds, and our world is busy. In the past, we were focused only on treating patients properly with surgery. Now we're asked to join in and help with the broader health issues. First you think, I'm already busy, and you wonder whether you'll find the time. But as our leader, Jeff, kept saying, 'Prevention is what we're about, and everyone needs to join in.' It slowly filtered down. It's no longer just me and my silo. We need to be part of it. I can order preventive tests and identify care gaps. Why not? As long as I'm not overstepping my area of expertise, I'm comfortable."

Dr. Brian Nguyen, Physician Director of Clinical Strategic Goals Optimization

"Kaiser Permanente has done a great job of improving prevention system-wide. We have put in place work systems for screening and preventing or slowing disease and morbidity. With the EMR, the speed of medicine has changed. We get instant feedback from the labs. Specialists may see the patient the same day I see them and we can communicate in real time. In the past there was a delay. The system tells me all the things my diabetic patient needs—things that I have to deal with today that used to happen over several months. We provide much better care, but there is more psychological stress on the physicians. We still are figuring out what this means for the amount of support and the amount of time we have with patients."

needs are being met. We can then spend more time evaluating their health status, diagnosing and treating disease, and working with patients to accelerate their recuperation and maintain the best possible levels of functioning. At SCPMG, we refer to that as "physicians doing physicians' work." And yet, we have to recognize that no matter how much support we provide, this increased emphasis on prevention does carry with it a broader set of responsibilities for all of our doctors. We have to recalibrate our expectations of our physicians, carefully document the impact of this focus not only on patients, but also on physicians, and align the incentives in the organization with this preventive focus.

Preventing and Slowing the Progression of Chronic Diseases

Prevention does not stop with screening and early detection—it continues to be an important orientation for us throughout the disease cycle. Chronic medical conditions are intimately tied up with prevention because so many chronic conditions are preventable! Chronic diseases—including cardiovascular disease, stroke, cancer, chronic obstructive pulmonary disease (COPD), diabetes, obesity, arthritis, and mouth and throat diseases–account for seven out of ten deaths in the US.[10] The CDC says that nearly 50 percent of the US adult population already suffers from at least one chronic condition.[11] Chronic disease is the US's "new epidemic" and already accounts for 78 percent of the costs in the healthcare system.[12]

This is happening for a variety of reasons including the lifestyle issues already discussed. People are living longer, and as they age generally have more medical issues, and develop more chronic conditions. As the approximately seventy-five million American baby boomers retire, care for aging populations is only going to become a larger issue within healthcare in the foreseeable future.[13] The Affordable Care Act takes aim at chronic disease through education and public campaigns and through grants for specific health activities, including reducing chronic disease rates. It will also (section 4108) implement Medicaid incentives to attack chronic diseases such as obesity, smoking, and diabetes.[14] Healthcare systems all over the world are implementing new approaches to deal with chronic illness, and many US systems, including Kaiser Permanente, were already experimenting with fundamental change in this area.[15]

Many healthcare systems have embarked on very systematic chronic disease management programs. For example, Minnesota-based HealthPartners has developed a system to track its 1.3 million members' health status and provide services dependent on their health status. They have applied extensive outreach, access to behavioral coaches, on-site workplace screenings and intensive disease and case management programs. These approaches are credited with preventing fourteen hundred condition specific events that would have required hospitalization, with 58 percent fewer hospitalization admissions for asthma and a 55 percent lower incidence of diabetes among program participants.[16] Utah-based Intermountain Healthcare has a number of clinical programs for chronic disease. These include a diabetes program that is spearheaded by a cross-discipline team, which includes endocrinologists, primary care doctors, nurses, pharmacists, and others. The program includes five areas of emphasis (see sidebar).[17]

It is essential that we closely manage chronic diseases with discipline and focus. Consider the patient with hypertension. Over six hundred thousand of our more than three million members are hypertensive. We not only measure but also treat aggressively. Eight years ago KPSC embarked on a program to measure blood pressure at every patient visit, in all departments, and to aggressively treat hypertension. This has allowed us to be the national leader in the HEDIS measures of blood pressure control in the Medicare population. If not adequately treated, hypertension results in multiple medical complications that we are aware of. In a similar vein, let's not forget diabetics, a challenging cohort of patients who require an eagle's eye watching over their medical care. By careful disease management, we have improved control of hemoglobin A1cs

Intermountain Healthcare's Diabetes Program

Intermountain Healthcare: A nonprofit health system with 28,000 employees, 21 hospitals, 600 employed physicians and a health plan that insures 500,000 people. Twenty-five percent of patients are insured by Intermountain.

Diabetes Program:

Led by the Intermountain Diabetes Team, including primary care physicians, endocrinologists, pharmacists, nurses, health plan care management leaders, and data management.

Includes 5 areas of emphasis:

- **Provider Education** including Clinical Education days that qualify for CME credit and are associated with incentive pay
- **Patient Education** including written material and qualified, reimbursable outpatient education often in primary care clinics.
- **Diabetes Patient Registries.** Each physician provided with quarterly list of patients with diabetes and summary of overall testing and control rates. Improvement is tied to incentives.
- **Clinical Support.** EMR with 21 key questions to ask of all diabetic patients, patient worksheets, and decision support.
- **Comprehensive Care.** Involvement of formulary, provision of health coaches and care managers.

Sample Results over a 9 year period: Significant improvement in A1c testing rates (from 79%→ 90%), 80% have hemoglobin A1c under 8; LDL testing improved from 67% to 87%; Blood pressure under 130 has increased from 43 to 55% of patients.

Source: Steven Towner, "Chronic Disease Management at Intermountain Healthcare," *Frontiers of Health Services Management.* 25, no. 2 (Winter 2008): 3-14.

and increased by 12.5 percent the number of diabetics whose HbA1c is less than 9. Diabetic lipid control has been improved as well.

At KPSC, as in other systems that are aggressively managing chronic disease, we enter data on our patients with chronic conditions into treatment registries and follow their diseases. Nurses help physicians manage these patients and their records. Our doctors and nurses send people who have diabetes, hypertension, COPD, and other chronic diseases to classes to educate them, so they can be armed with sound knowledge to better control their disease. Education is cost effective and it makes a difference, and we incorporate it into care as much as possible.[18] We have made it easier for patients to be educated by launching online education programs. We have made it as easy as possible for physicians to "write a prescription" for a weight loss or smoking cessation class, which will link a patient with health coaches who are trained to deal with the particular condition. By providing these supplemental resources, we try not to saddle doctors with a lot more work, but to make us part of an extended team, each reinforcing the messages provided by the others. Effective prevention takes time—time spent in conversations with patients, and time checking to make sure that, for example, the patient is indeed walking at lunch and diligently controlling his diabetes.

Physicians need to be a voice for building healthcare systems that have these resources, and then for working in concert with them. It would be easy enough to say "Isn't that the patient's responsibility?" and fundamentally it is. And yet we know that if we don't provide support and encouragement, we will, as a society, lose the battle to build a sustainable health system. We will become overwhelmed by the costs that are incurred in a system plagued by unnecessary flare-ups of disease, needless hospitalizations, and other heroic emergency interventions that can result in a continuous drain on our time and energies. And we will have let our patients down because we haven't done all that we can to keep them healthy.

Prevention is clearly powerful, but it changes a lot of relationships, and that can be very unsettling. We need to be part of a team. Many are now concluding that nurse practitioners and physician assistants are the natural go-to people for this kind of care because physicians are too busy, and indeed KPSC has created many specialized roles for coaching, monitoring and educating. Yet, according to Nancy Spiegel, our head of Leadership and Organizational Development, who has been centrally involved in designing many of these support programs, "We've made it easier through the Proactive Office Encounter [POE] and the medical record, and the systems we've set up for physicians to refer patients to these specialized support groups. But if the physician raises the issue and says 'go here for help,' the patient is more likely to do it."

Responsibility for prevention has to extend to a much larger segment of employees in the healthcare system who now have to work together in a coordinated way: nurses, PAs, doctors, pharmacists, and administrative staff. Furthermore, modern communications technology is making it easier to monitor the health status of chronically ill patients, even in their own homes, and to provide them with automatic reminders of the steps they need to take to keep their condition under control. The patient and her family become part of the healthcare team! Yet that doesn't let us off the hook. Our patients will continue to look to their physicians for support and guidance.

Preventing Adverse Outcomes in the Hospitalized Patient

The fourth preventive prescription is to ensure the safety of those who end up in a hospital bed despite all our best intentions and medical skill. Yearly, more than ninety-eight thousand patients die in US hospitals from iatrogenic causes such as adverse drug interactions, hospital-acquired infections, and surgical mishaps.[19] Having an EMR certainly helps, by calling out drugs that are contraindicated because of allergy or potential interaction with other drugs, and by drawing attention to related aspects of a patient's medical history. Although we do not control all the processes and procedures followed in our hospitals, we physicians need to lead the care of our hospitalized patients with a focus on preventing unnecessary negative outcomes. We need to be a voice to ensure that the processes followed in hospitals are systematic, coordinated, and efficient. No one wants to be in the hospital longer than necessary, and the best way to get patients home quickly is to give them integrated, safe, care.

In the KPSC system, the medical group (SCPMG) and the hospitals (the Kaiser Foundation Hospitals, or KFH) have worked together to develop specific initiatives to combat hospital-acquired infections and other hospital-acquired conditions. We have especially targeted catheter-induced blood stream infections, pressure ulcers, retained foreign objects, surgical site infections for hip and knee replacements, and ventilator-induced pneumonias. Each of these initiatives, with ongoing senior leadership support from both SCPMG and the hospitals, is championed by a physician and a non-physician acting as a team on the local level. The champions also are charged with sharing best practices, internally and externally, and are jointly accountable for progress toward the agreed-upon goals, tracking progress and quickly identifying root causes and implementing process changes where needed. We are proud of the progress we have made, which has kept us below the California and national averages in these areas.

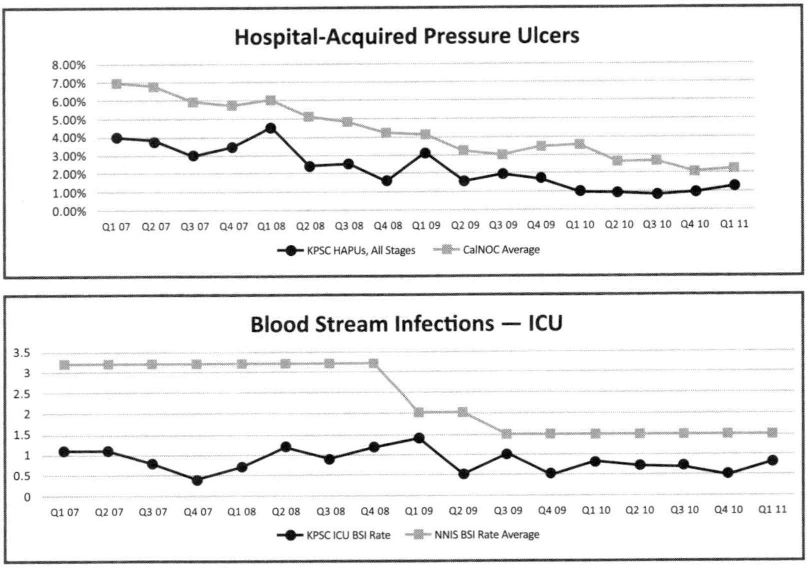

Figure 4: *Hospital Patient Safety Measures Improvement*

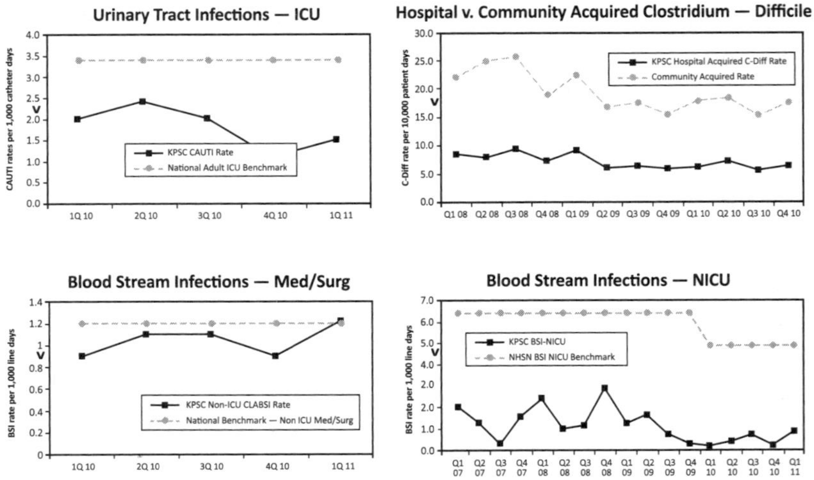

Figure 5: *Hospital Infection Control Improvement*
(Note: The national benchmark in the Blood Stream Infections-NICU graph was lowered in 2010.)

The hospitals' unit-based teams (UBTs) continually focus on pressure ulcers, recognizing that they add unnecessary complications to what is already a very complicated job. Multiple interventions are done in the course of a hospitalization, beginning with a skin assessment upon admission to a hospital unit. Unit-based teams are a key component of our approach. They are defined in the 2005 National Agreement between the Coalition of Kaiser Permanente Unions and Kaiser Foundation Health Plan, Kaiser Foundation Hospitals and the Permanente Medical Groups. This is an approach to work that gives front-line supervisors and staff responsibility and accountability for continually improving service in the system.[20] Our physicians support these teams and are expected to be vigilant about patient safety and to provide leadership to ensure these measures are tracked and improved.

Conscientious care doesn't stop at the door to the hospital. Patients want a clear sense of what they can and should do to continue their recovery process at home. The concept of transitional care is gaining traction in many care settings and systems as a way to bridge the gap and deliver continuity of care as our patients move from facility to home or to other healthcare settings.[21] American hospitals' readmission rates are a critical issue. Unplanned readmission occurs in 20 percent of all Medicare patients in the US.[22] The monitoring done by such groups as the National Healthcare Safety Network (NHSN), National Nosocomial Infections Surveillance (NNIS), and Collaborative Alliance for Nursing Outcomes (CALNOC) has provided a big push to increase safety and reduce readmissions rates. Systems all over the country are working on these factors.

One exemplary program is at the Group Health Cooperative in Seattle. It has decreased hospital readmissions to 12 percent through its Emergency Department and Hospital Inpatient Improvement Program, by systematically focusing on smooth and safe transitions out of the hospital (see sidebar).[23] Comprehensive discharge processes are essential. In order to provide the best possible care for our patients, we physicians need to play an active role in making sure it is happening. We can't say, "That's not our job."

Our Own Wellness: Setting the Stage for a Prevention-Focused Healthcare System

To build wellness and prevention into the healthcare delivery system, the entire healthcare workforce, physicians and non-physicians alike, needs to focus on their own health and wellness. As employers and companies wrestle

Transition Care Improvement at Group Health Cooperative

- A Seattle-based, consumer-governed, nonprofit health care system that coordinates care and coverage for 600,000 residents of Washington and Idaho.
- Care is delivered by subsidiary carriers, Group Health Options, Inc. and KPS Health Plans.

Readmission Medicare Rate

- Has fallen from 16% to 12%, far below the 20% national average

The Improvement Process

- Used the Lean Methodology to redesign four subprocesses, including admissions, involved in transition out of the hospital
- Involved front-line clinical staff, including hospitalists, medical directors, administrative managers, and clinical managers

New Transition Processes Include

- Teaming between case managers, physicians and ED staff to ensure that patients are not admitted inappropriately, and get help to transition directly to the best care setting.
- Daily huddles of hospitalists and case managers to discuss each patient and plan in advance for effective and safe transition
- High touch care coordination with three chair-side visits from care managers who teach patients about their diagnoses, medicines and post-discharge care
- Contact within forty-eight hours with patients with complex medical needs to answer questions, discuss medication procedures and schedule follow-up care

Source: Alliance of Community Health Plans, *Investing in Outcomes. Creating Value: Group Health* (n.d.), http://www.achp.org/files.php?force&file=/ACHP_GroupHealth_CaseStudy_932428296.pdf.

with the cost of healthcare, they have started to address the health of their own workers. The healthcare industry is beginning to set the example and lead the way. The Cleveland Clinic, for example, no longer hires smokers.[24] It has also removed all trans-fats from its cafeterias.[25] Indiana University Health (formerly Clarian Health Partners) incentivizes its workers with additional pay when they meet specified health targets through its Wellness Track plan.[26] Many hospitals, including Geisinger Health System, Johns Hopkins Health System, and the Cook County Health & Hospitals System, mandate receiving the influenza vaccine for employees (although there is some allowance for exceptions).[27]

Healthy workers have increased productivity and are less likely to come to work sick, as compared to those workers with risk factors and poor health. *Zero Trends* author Dee Edington provides examples of companies where for employees who completed health risk assessments (HRAs), healthcare costs escalated only one third as quickly as for other employees who did not complete the assessment.[28] Following up on the assessment with biometric screenings and prevention initiatives, along with onsite coaching at work, is shown to result in healthier and more productive employees. Similarly, health promotion initiatives based on health risk assessments have been shown to save hundreds of dollars a year per participant in a population of Medicare beneficiaries. [29] These same benefits should also accrue to healthcare employees when we focus on our own health and wellness.

I mentioned earlier that two-thirds of workers today are overweight. That's true no matter what company employs them. The healthcare profession is not immune to this problem. There is an urgent need to reverse this trend and the risk factors and disease that will eventually ensue. At SCPMG we are working to create a culture where our physicians and the entire health team address our own health—which both allows us to be good role models, and to be more persuasive in our conversations with patients about these issues. We will also come to work better able to provide high-quality care to our patients and healthcare members. We have moved forward with multiple initiatives, including doing away with sugar-laden soft drinks in our cafeterias, and campaigns for everyone to take the stairs and walk on wellness trails around our campuses. We sponsor fitness challenges in the workplace, as well as marathons and triathlons in the community. We have taken Kaiser Permanente's "Thrive" brand to heart.

Going forward, SCPMG is creating a pilot program to encourage employees to pay more attention to their health and wellness. The pilot allows employees to get credits that add value to their fringe benefit plan for meeting certain objectives, like taking a total health assessment, getting a flu shot, or taking an online health education program at our kp.org portal. Physicians have been active in crafting all of these programs and are frequent participants in many of the initiatives. Our employees are our patients and co-workers. We benefit from providing care to a healthier population, working with healthier people, and being healthier ourselves—a true win-win-win proposition.

Prevention: How We Assess Our Impact

By broadening our perspective, we physicians can enhance our contribution to the society and populations we serve. This does not imply abandoning our traditional focus on treating illness, repairing injury, restoring health, and preventing suffering. Rather, it is a shift to think about our role in terms of our impact on people's overall health status and quality of life, and to play an active leadership role in preventing and slowing the progression of disease. As Nancy Spiegel points out, "Physicians still have the same core identity—to treat illness. But they're realizing that there are a lot of people coming to see them whose illnesses and flare-ups are a result of lifestyle. Physicians can help these people best by encouraging them to do the things necessary to stay out of their office." It is only through such an emphasis that society will be able and willing to continue to pay the costs for our services. This challenges all of us, personally and as a team with our colleagues and co-workers, to deliver on the promise of the medical profession to society. I believe this will restore the luster of our profession, in our own and others' eyes.

An approach to healthcare based on prevention puts a lot of weight on outcomes, especially the lack of manifestation of disease. Indeed, medical reimbursement processes seem to be slowly moving toward this target. It's a big change, and it may make us extremely nervous. How do you get paid for something that doesn't ever manifest? How are our services valued? How do we get recognition for the surgery that was averted? We have to make sure we are at the table and playing a leadership role in how this will happen, so that we can continue to have professional careers where we can practice medicine successfully, with high quality, and with great pride. I'll talk more about outcomes, and value, and the new standards of accountability in chapter five.

Trend	Implications for Physicians	Am I effectively dealing with this trend now?
Move Upstream in the Disease Cycle to Concentrate on Prevention		
	1. Take a broad view of patients and consider their total wellness, not just diseases. 2. Legislation and reimbursement trends will force increased focus on prevention and outcomes. Eventually reimbursements will be tied to outcomes. 3. Pay attention to lifestyle issues such as smoking, drinking, and obesity, which continue to impact large numbers of patients. 4. Flexible and timely approaches to treat acute illness or injury	
Integrated Healthcare Teams		
	1. Prevention is the responsibility of all of us. We are part of a team. 2. Other team members, such as nurses, office staff, and physician assistants, will support us in managing prevention goals in a comprehensive way.	
Chronic Diseases		
	1. We are part of the team having to deal with the huge incidence of chronic diseases. 2. Care of patients with chronic conditions will be increasingly managed with the help of registries. 3. We will pay more attention to patient education and connecting patients to appropriate resources.	

Trend	Implications for Physicians	Am I effectively dealing with this trend now?
Iatrogenic Disease and Post-Hospital Care		
	1. Safety is our responsibility too. 2. We will actively influence the hospital procedures/ process to avoid hospital-acquired infections and conditions. 3. We have a role to play in focusing on post-discharge treatment to decrease unplanned readmissions.	
Healthcare Professionals Need to Be Healthy, Too		
	1. We will set an example for the rest of society and focus on our own health and wellness. 2. We will make sure we and other healthcare professionals work in healthy environments.	

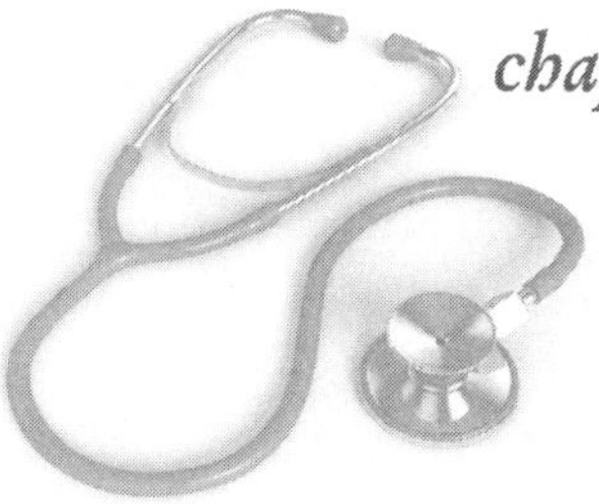

chapter three

Patient-Centered Care

It is not possible to overestimate the importance of the patient-centered movement in healthcare. The service we provide is not an impersonal, mechanical, transactional set of activities where we simply interpret a test, diagnose an illness, write a prescription, perform a surgical operation, and respond to patients and conditions that present themselves. We can bring the highest level of technical expertise, medical knowledge, and beautifully engineered and efficient processes to our work, but if we do not put the patient at the center of our attention and ensure that she or he has a positive experience, we simply do not deliver good healthcare. Our expertise must include the ability to create an experience for each patient that leads to the best possible outcomes. A patient-centered focus results in not only improving the doctor-patient relationship but also in improving quality outcomes.[1]

My views on patient-centered care are based on my thirty years of experience caring for patients as an internist with a subspecialty in hematology oncology. As a cancer physician, I saw that the keys to success started with an accurate diagnosis and timely treatment; but just as important was bonding with patients through empathy and honest and respectful interactions. That's why service is the area I am most passionate about. If you're a really intelligent doctor but don't care about the patient, I would not want to hire you into our system. I wouldn't want you as my personal physician or my family's physician, either!

The field we work in is unique. When people become "patients" and interact with us, they very well may be going through some of the most poignant times of their lives: possibly the happiest, possibly the most intensely sorrowful. We assist a woman in bringing a much-desired child into the world, and we are also there when a car crash victim breathes his last breath. We stand with the person whose elderly parent has just died. And yes, we are there in patients' lives at more mundane times too. But in general, we touch people's lives at times when they are physically vulnerable, emotionally exposed, facing unknowns great and small, and in need of help. This is not just a job; medicine is a calling.

We all know that patients with similar presenting symptoms can have radically different outcomes depending upon their behavior. Some of these behaviors include adherence, attitude, levels of anxiety, levels of comprehension of their situation, and whether or not they take responsibility for their own health. By paying attention to a patient's emotional and psychological state and by carefully designing the therapeutic environment, we can positively influence the patient's orientation towards healing and health.

Historically, our profession did not think about interactions with patients this way. Instead, we were focused on the disease and the disease agent. Or perhaps we doctors put ourselves in the center of focus. I think we can admit that everything used to be arranged according to the convenience of the doctors, and secondarily to the other members of the healthcare team. But that is truly changing. Healthcare, as we discussed in the last chapter, is moving from a narrow focus on disease toward embracing wellness. Doctors are similarly enlarging our focus to include not only the disease itself or our own needs as doctors, but also the patient's needs and perspective. Now many healthcare systems are redesigning themselves to put the patient in the middle, which will provide even greater support for patient-centric medicine.

When I assumed the role of executive medical director of SCPMG in 2004, I was determined to emphasize service. I made it clear that all patients, no matter whom they see or where they are, should receive exceptional care and have a positive experience when interacting with anyone in our system. Service is much more than the doctor, nurse, and receptionist being considerate of patients. Patient-centered care also should focus on the "aesthetics" of the experience for patients, that is, how they experience our services and how they feel about the care. Do they understand the experience? Does it make sense to them? Are their needs being met? Does it fit into their life context? Do we set up positive emotions and pleasant sensory connections at the various touch points? Is the experience user-friendly and convenient? Patients are the consumers or users of our medical services. To truly be patient-centric, we must effectively address their goals, needs, and preferences for the experience.[2]

Creating a Caring Environment

Be a patient for a minute: you have decided you need to see a doctor. You're worried. You called the doctor's office over the weekend and got an answering machine. You didn't think it was an emergency, so you waited to talk to someone on Monday. You get an appointment but you have to cancel an important meeting in order to fit the time slot. If you're visiting a new doctor or this is a new ailment, you may not know what to expect at the office visit. If it is your first visit to a specific office or medical center, you then have to figure out driving directions. Is it easy to find the building you're supposed to go to, or do you have to drive around the block a couple of times, straining to see building signage? Where do you park? Are you running late? You may feel like a nervous wreck. Sometimes you can't even figure out how to navigate through the building to the correct department. Have you ever had to sit for so long in a waiting room that you begin to think you're invisible? All of these little aggravations and indignities are piled on top of the worries about your health condition—and you haven't even seen the doctor yet! These are some examples of what patients go through so that we healthcare professionals can see them at our convenience. In contrast, being patient-centered means creating experiences that minimize fear, anxiety, confusion, uncertainty, and panic.

Does it really surprise anyone that clinics in retail stores are becoming more popular? They are starting to pop up in drug stores, such as the MinuteClinics in CVS stores, which are generally open seven days a week and some evenings. The MinuteClinic website lists actual prices (e.g., DTaP vaccination, $99.99 in California) along with the insurance plans that will pay for visits.[3] No appointment is needed. The clinics are in places where patients go in their everyday lives. They can get in and out quickly. Just the fact that these clinics are open on the weekend is a major revelation. Who mandated that people can only get sick during the week?

The place where many of us spend most of our waking hours is also starting to house healthcare, that is, at the workplace. We're seeing more and more workplace health clinics that offer a range of services, including preventive care, wellness services, occupational health, acute care, and disease management.[4] Large and even small companies are partnering with healthcare organizations to operate joint clinics. Cisco Systems's LifeConnections Health Center at its headquarters campus in San Jose, California, is one example. It includes primary care, laboratory, radiology, vision care, chiropractic, and disease management services. The company also has a fitness center and a day care center onsite, as well as a Walgreen's pharmacy. Physicians from three healthcare plans, Kaiser Permanente, Cigna, and UnitedHealthcare, work onsite. These medical services are very popular with Cisco employees. Forty-three percent of eligible employees use them, and 83 percent of employees see this as a valuable benefit. Cisco offers telemedicine services to employees at other sites as far away as North Carolina. As a result, it reports productivity gains and cost savings.[5]

Onsite medical care is certainly much more convenient for workers. There is almost no travel time involved, so there is much less time away from work. This is a nice incentive for companies paying a large share of the costs of healthcare and enduring the loss of productivity resulting from employee trips to the doctor. In a bid to offer an additional way of taking care to our patients instead of making them come to us, KPSC operates a mobile health clinic van that goes out to our members' workplaces.[6] We are piloting workplace clinics and are exploring other ways to bring healthcare to the work setting. This means some physicians will be practicing medicine in different settings—on the patient's turf, not ours.

Service is Now Viewed as an Entitlement

Patients are rightly expecting more than they used to from their healthcare experiences. And they no longer have unquestioning respect for our judgment, motives, or for the confusing and byzantine processes we may have in our offices and hospitals. Understandably, patients can get rather irritated when they have to fill out the same paperwork every time they come in to see the same doctor. When the specialist doesn't have the results from the test that was conducted last week, patients know the system is being inefficient and is failing them. Knowledgeable patients know when the physician is not taking the time to discuss options of care with them.

We have to earn the respect of our patients not only for our clinical prowess, but also for the experience they have using our services, and their trust that we are operating in their best interests, not ours. Service expectations in today's world are high and growing. Yelp and Angie's List are just two of the many websites where prospective patients can read reviews of the experience that others have had with particular doctors. With the Internet, if we deliver subpar service, the world will know with a click of a button.

At KPSC, our journey to become a service-oriented culture has been eye-opening for all of us. We had always been known for giving good technical care at a reasonable price, but also for mediocre service. In recent years, we have put a much more robust focus on the patient-care experience. As we have done so, our reputation for more personalized, patient-focused service has positively affected the morale and pride of our physicians, other providers, and the administrative staff, not to mention the attitudes of our members. Our doctors are very proud to say they deliver care at KP.

Changing the organizational culture to achieve an excellent service reputation has been a huge and ongoing effort. The letters we receive, such as the one below, let us see whether we're succeeding in creating the service experience the patient values. We regularly share feedback, whether positive or negative, with our staff. Our approach has been to make the coordination of care across our system everyone's responsibility. Patient satisfaction is everyone's goal.

June 28, 2011

To Several Kaiser Permanente Executives

Dear Gentlemen:

I have been a satisfied Kaiser subscriber for a number of years, but my most recent experience, at a time when I had a serious medical issue, was so overwhelmingly positive that I wanted to bring it to your attention.

Over the weekend of May 14-15 this year, I began to experience vision problems that ultimately proved to be because of a detached retina in my right eye. First thing the following Monday I e-mailed my primary care physician at the Thousand Oaks office seeking advice and an appointment. Her schedule was fully booked that day, but with the help of her staff I saw another doctor at eleven o'clock the same morning. He examined me and immediately called an ophthalmologist at Woodland Hills seeking a same day appointment for me with her. I saw her at two o'clock that afternoon. She examined me and immediately called the eye surgeon at Panorama City. They discussed my symptoms, now diagnosed as a detached retina, and he inquired if I was on blood thinners (I am on an aspirin regimen).

Because of that, the earliest we could do the requisite surgery was that Thursday evening. He examined me on Wednesday and advised me to come to the hospital there on Thursday, which I did.

A lot had to happen that day. I needed blood tests and an EKG prior to surgery and to complete the paperwork for admission and report to pre-op. In all, I had to visit six different entities at the hospital to get all of this done. I was amazed that all of the tests and paperwork were completed in two hours and fifteen minutes! (Within an hour, I received the results of my blood tests on my iPhone!) At every station, I was greeted courteously. Every Kaiser staff member I dealt with that day was friendly, efficient, professional, and clearly interested in seeing that I had a quality experience at the hospital. Regrettably, I did not have the chance to record all of their names, but I do want to recognize and thank:

- Dr. Joni Jordan, my primary care physician, at Thousand Oaks
- LVN Dawn Groom at Thousand Oaks
- LVN Griselda Orozco at Thousand Oaks
- Dr. Eduard Osmonov at Thousand Oaks
- Dr. Patricia Shih-Chia Tsai at Woodland Hills
- Dr. Navid Khodadadi at Panorama City and his nurse
- The receptionist in Ophthalmology, PEEK, and elsewhere
- The EKG technician and the phlebotomist
- The nurses and support staff in pre-op
- Dr. Khodadadi's surgical team
- The bevy of other staff members who worked with me and for me that day.

You have assembled a first class team of medical practitioners and support staff. It is even more impressive that all of the staff manifest such a positive, affirmative organization culture. Every staff member I encountered was "tuned in and turned on" to seeing that the patient had a positive experience. That is impressive.

You all have my sincere thanks and appreciation.

Charles Maxey
Thousand Oaks, CA

Figure 1: *Letter from Charles Maxey, KP Patient*

If service problems exist in an integrated system like Kaiser Permanente, they can be magnified in a fragmented system where patients are shuttled from office to office and facility to facility. In fact, a 2010 Commonwealth Fund study of the perceptions of both physicians and patients in seven countries found that compared to the others, the US is perceived by its stakeholders as being in the middle of the pack at providing effective and patient-centered care, but only fifth or lower in providing safe, coordinated, timely, and efficient care, and in contributing to patients leading long, healthy and productive lives.[7]

Country Rankings	
	1.00–2.33
	2.34–4.66
	4.67–7.00

	AUS	CAN	GER	NETH	NZ	UK	US
OVERALL RANKING (2010)	3	6	4	1	5	2	7
Quality Care	4	7	5	2	1	3	6
Effective Care	2	7	6	3	5	1	4
Safe Care	6	5	3	1	4	2	7
Coordinated Care	4	5	7	2	1	3	6
Patient-Centered Care	2	5	3	6	1	7	4
Access	6.5	5	3	1	4	2	6.5
Cost-Related Problem	6	3.5	3.5	2	5	1	7
Timeliness of Care	6	7	2	1	3	4	5
Efficiency	2	6	5	3	4	1	7
Equity	4	5	3	1	6	2	7
Long, Healthy, Productive Lives	1	2	3	4	5	6	7
Health Expenditures/Capita, 2007	$3,357	$3,895	$3,588	$3,837*	$2,454	$2,992	$7,290

Note: * Estimate. Expenditures shown in $US PPP (purchasing power parity).
Source: Calculated by The Commonwealth Fund based on 2007 International Health Policy Survey; 2008 International Health Policy Survey of Sicker Adults; 2009 International Health Policy Survey of Primary Care Physicians; Commonwealth Fund Commission on a High Performance Health System National Scorecard; and Organization for Economic Cooperation and Development, *OECD Health Data, 2009* (Paris: OECD, Nov. 2009).

THE COMMONWEALTH FUND

Figure 2: *Comparing the US Healthcare System to Healthcare in Six Other Countries.*
Source: Karen Davis, Cathy Schoen, and Kristof Stremikis, Mirror, Mirror on the Wall: How the Performance of the US Healthcare System Compares Internationally, 2010 Update *(June 2010), http://www.commonwealthfund.org/Content/Publications/Fund-Reports/2010/Jun/Mirror-Mirror-Update.aspx?page=all. Reprinted by permission.*

The travesty is that poor care experiences negatively affect patient outcomes, undermine our mission in healthcare, and defeat our purposes as physicians. It is not just that people don't *think* they receive good quality healthcare if they don't have a good patient experience. It's that they really don't. The frustrations experienced while trying to get needed care can be very stressful. We are becoming increasingly aware in the medical community of the negative impact of stress on health status. We certainly should not be perpetuating dissatisfying healthcare encounters that work against our mission to improve the health of our patients.

We have done a great many things across the KPSC system, including seemingly simple things, as well as substantial innovations, to put a laser-like focus on the patient care experience. Taken together, these add up to a more positive experience for the patient. For one thing, we're carefully tracking how patients are experiencing their care, and targeting areas that they think are important. And we're tracking and making steady progress against regional and national standards.

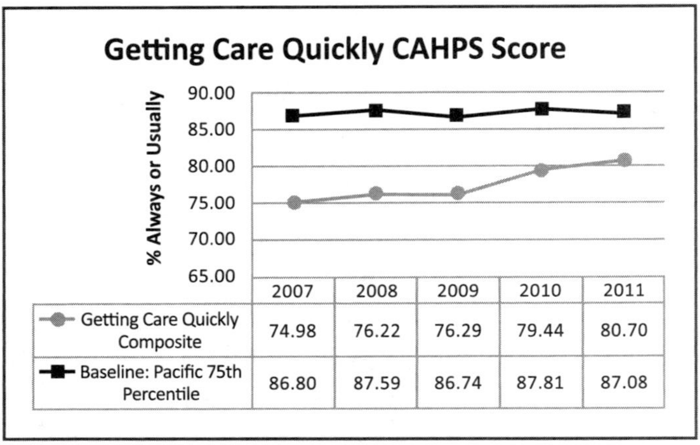

	2007	2008	2009	2010	2011
Getting Care Quickly Composite	74.98	76.22	76.29	79.44	80.70
Baseline: Pacific 75th Percentile	86.80	87.59	86.74	87.81	87.08

Figure 3: *Consumer Assessment of Healthcare Providers and Systems (CAHPS) 2007–2011 KPSC Trend Data on Getting Care Quickly*

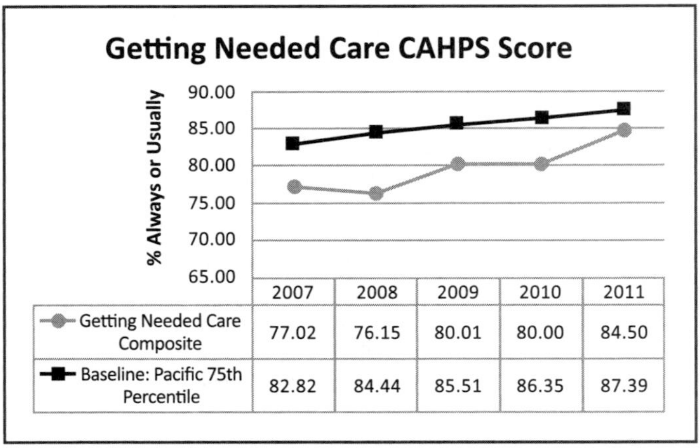

	2007	2008	2009	2010	2011
Getting Needed Care Composite	77.02	76.15	80.01	80.00	84.50
Baseline: Pacific 75th Percentile	82.82	84.44	85.51	86.35	87.39

Figure 4: *Consumer Assessment of Healthcare Providers and Systems (CAHPS) 2007–2011 KPSC Trend Data on Getting Needed Care*

First, there are the little things that mean a lot. Most KPSC facilities have self-service kiosks where patients can check in for their appointments and pay. These are just like the kiosks at the airport and reduce the time spent waiting in line. At our large and sprawling Los Angeles Medical Center on Sunset Boulevard, the outside building signage is oversize, very visible, and easily readable. This ensures that patients don't have to drive or walk around in circles trying to find the correct building in this high-density, high-traffic section of the city. In each of our exam rooms, we have installed special screensavers so patients can enjoy a diversion that will possibly educate them on health and relevant information while waiting for the doctor. As an option instead of an in-person tour, expectant parents can go online and take virtual OB tours of KPSC birthing facilities.[8] Each location has a webpage with several 360 degree views, including the facility exterior, the delivery suite, the nursery, and a patient room, plus phone numbers and directions.

We work hard to ensure timely access to care, because reducing wait times is a patient satisfier, a clear indication that we are respectful of the patient's time, and contributes to high-quality care. New members can call for wellness exam appointments that will be scheduled within thirty days of the request. Our target for a specialty appointment is nine days or fewer. If a patient needs additional tests and is already at a facility, we strive to get the additional tests done on the same day. This prevents a second trip and an inconvenience to the patient. Before new mothers leave the hospital, we have already scheduled their first post-delivery appointment, which is usually within a week. The visit generally includes a meeting with a lactation consultant.

We all know how incredibly irritating long automated phone trees are and how they waste our time. Real people answer our phones, and we're committed to making this happen in a timely fashion. And it is understood that answers to patients' questions will be forthcoming in an equally timely manner. Losing phone messages or not returning phone calls is never OK.

Communication—the Sine Qua Non of High-Quality Healthcare

It goes without saying that communication and language are critical to the delivery of medical services and strongly related to patient understanding and adherence to the treatment plan. Language barriers may lead to errors in diagnosis and treatment. Equally important, communication problems can be a serious impediment to trust.[9] In California, 39.5 percent of the population speaks a primary language other than English.[10] In Southern

California, Spanish is the second most-spoken language. As mandated by law,[11] KPSC has interpreters for patients who are seen by doctors who don't speak their language. But we strongly believe that higher quality and more equitable care is delivered when doctors have the language capability to speak directly with their patients. Toward this goal, we have implemented a language concordance program, matching non-English speaking patients with bilingual doctors who speak their language. When we started the program, only 26 percent of the visits by our Limited English Proficient patients (88 percent Spanish-speaking) were with a bilingual physician. I am proud that we have improved the rate to 36 percent and are now expanding the program to our specialty physicians.

Dr. Patricia De La Riva is a pediatrician at the KPSC Woodland Hills Medical Center. She is a Culturally Responsive Care Physician Champion and a Language Concordance Physician Champion and is fluent in English and Spanish. Pediatricians not only deal with patients (children), but with their families, and Dr. De La Riva believes that developing trusting relationships is especially critical for good pediatric care. Of the twenty-four hundred patients in her panel, about 21 percent of them speak only Spanish. Language skills and awareness of cultural complexities are keys to effectively developing that relationship. She notes, "I believe I gain trust and develop a better relationship with a Spanish-speaking family quicker than an English-speaking physician who is struggling to use an interpreter (face-to-face) or the language line." On a practical level, language concordance enables better history taking and compliance. De La Riva sees it as a powerful tool for providing good, consistent, quality care.

Doctors have to pass a certified test to be part of the language concordance program. For those interested physicians who would like to increase their language proficiency in Spanish, we provide Rosetta Stone language training. Physicians brushing up on their Spanish skills can also attend a four-week language immersion program in Costa Rica or Mexico, which includes a clinical component.

The importance of genuine communication between patient and physician can't be overemphasized. We recognize that some physicians may have personal and political beliefs regarding the obligation to accommodate non-English speaking people living and receiving care in the United States. Yet we live in a world that is increasingly global and in societies that are increasingly multi-cultural and multi-lingual. It *is* our obligation to deliver excellent healthcare and service to any person who walks through our doors. Our medical director for Quality and Clinical Analysis, Dr. Michael Kanter, notes that despite all of our fancy medical technology, "The old-fashioned Marcus Welby talking-to-the-patient approach is often what makes the difference." [12] If you are hindered by language, your ability to relate to the patient and build rapport is compromised. Each of us may not have the obligation to learn to conduct our work in other languages, but as a profession we certainly have the obligation to make sure that we can provide high-quality healthcare for all.

The language issue of patient-centric care goes further. Even native English speaking patients experience language—or at least understanding—barriers. We physicians go rapidly through information and terminology that to us is second nature but is often incomprehensible to a patient. If we're a cardiologist helping our patient deal with heart failure, for example, we're personally on familiar territory, but how much of what we say is really understood by a layperson? How little salt for a "low-salt diet"? What is "too much" fluid? What does it mean that someone might retain fluid? What does it mean that a heart is beating irregularly, and how dangerous is it? We have to remember that for each patient this is likely to be the first visit to a strange land.

Going through things once, verbally, is not enough for most patients. At KPSC, after every appointment, we give our patients a written After Visit Summary. It summarizes the appointment and the diagnosis, prescriptions for drugs, behavioral lifestyle issues that have been mentioned, and explanations of what happens next. It also lists any future appointments and other comments by the physician. It may seem like a simple thing, but a written report is truly helpful. It's well-known that patients, particularly when anxious about their health, do not always process or remember what they are told during an appointment. This is especially true if they are hearing unfamiliar terms or getting complicated instructions.

Culturally Responsive Care

Culturally responsive care goes well beyond language. We must be cognizant of many factors when caring for patients who come from a different culture, race, ethnic group, or sexual orientation. Culture manifests itself in customs, beliefs, and values, among other things.[13] For example, although the Latino population is not a homogeneous group, there are some general themes that many Latinos share. Many of these are not in accordance with the dominant US cultural paradigm. These include concepts of family, respect, faith, and

"We're treating people, not arteries. Once you have a trusting relationship between doctor and patient–you can overcome some of the resistance to receiving care and the skepticism. Our doctors came up with a whole host of ways to build trusting relationships and to capitalize on these trusting relationships to improve health care outcomes."

– Dr. Howard Fullman, Area Medical Director of Kaiser Permanente West Los Angeles

fatalism, among others. The importance of family may be seen, for example, when a patient brings several family members along to a doctor visit. Latinos tend to respect people in authority, including physicians. This may be manifested by a patient not looking directly at the physician.[14] Doctors need to have adequate knowledge and understanding of cultural differences to successfully deliver quality care in these situations.

KPSC's West Los Angeles Medical Center is a Center for Excellence in African-American Health. The clinic has a special focus on disease and health conditions faced by African-Americans, most notably sickle cell disease, congestive heart failure, and prostate cancer.[15] Dr. Howard Fullman, area medical director of Kaiser Permanente West Los Angeles, notes that the focus started about a decade ago after a report from the Institute of Medicine found large disparities in care for minorities in our country compared to Caucasians.[16] The physicians and staff at the very diverse medical center started working hard to address this issue. With their initial focus on sickle cell disease, followed by a subsequent focus on additional conditions, the importance of trust, personalized care, and social support became salient. Care delivery and case management have to be led by highly empathetic physicians and staff. The medical center started embedding many aspects of personalization and empathy into the way they function, including sensitizing physicians to the issues of touch, respect, and personal concern in the physician/patient relationship. The Center found ways to personalize outreach and individualized educational interactions with patients. "We're treating people, not arteries," says Dr. Fullman. "Once you have a trusting relationship between doctor and patient—you can overcome some of the resistance to receiving care and the skepticism. Our doctors came up with a whole host of ways to build trusting relationships and to capitalize on these trusting relationships to improve healthcare outcomes." The health disparities between African-Americans and Caucasians at West Los Angeles are much lower than in the United States population at large or even in the rest of the KP population. And the outcomes are improving day-by-day; the trajectory is excellent. We are closing the gap to parity.

Individualizing Care

Patient-centered care entails increasingly more individualized care. This means aligning our diagnostic testing and treatment to the individual patient's risk factors, life context, overall health status, multiple conditions, demographics, and personal preferences. It means embracing the full variety of patients who come through our doors. It also means establishing a trust relationship and connections with patients to help them take care of themselves.

Proactive Care. Medicine has been a profession where we practice with an expectation that our patients come to us when they need something. If a patient chooses to come in for a yearly check-up, we conduct an exam, measure vital signs, look through the charts and recommend preventive and other measures. If the Federal Drug Administration (FDA) issues guidance on a drug or a device, doctors often hope that the patients to whom we have prescribed this drug or installed the device will reach out to us to find out what to do. We don't worry too much about the ones who don't come in. Yet we are aware that there are huge costs to society from untreated disease or diseases being diagnosed in their later stages and from failing to prevent unnecessary illness. As we know, survival rates for patients diagnosed with cancers, for example, vary greatly depending on when the cancer is caught, as does the economic cost.[17]

Patient-focused care is not passive care. We have to reach out to patients to make sure they are receiving the care necessary to get or stay healthy. This doesn't mean the physician does it all. Rather, it means the physician is a leader in a team that is centered around the patient. One major approach that we've instituted at SCPMG puts our focus squarely on patients: the Proactive Office Encounter (POE), in which all healthcare providers and support staff in the system have accountability to reach out to our patients to make sure they are accessing needed care. In addition, our registries and outreach enable us to reach patients who may not show up on our doorstep.

We instituted the POE to ensure our doctors have sufficient time to address preventive screenings. The national literature notes that a typical primary care physician caring for a panel of two thousand patients would have to work approximately eighteen hours a day to make sure that she provided the recommended preventive screenings and proper treatment of her patients' chronic diseases.[18] This would clearly be an untenable situation for our physicians, and a barrier to improving the health status of our members.

Therefore we have a created a system that focuses all of us on prevention and provides a support team for the physician. All of our patients' needs for preventive and chronic care are flagged in the EMR. All staff interacting with patients, including in our specialty offices, are charged with bringing unmet care needs to the attention of the patient and helping to arrange for appropriate care.

Creating Individualized Patient Pathways. In our medical practices we all see a wide variety of patients with quite different needs and preferences, and we can't approach all of our patients in the same way. Our systems need to be set up to handle many different kinds of care requirements that vary depending on the nature of the presenting problem and where the patient is along the health continuum. Our more fortunate patients are fundamentally healthy and need only occasional visits, but still need a focus on prevention. We have to be active in intervening with patients with risk factors and those who develop conditions such as hypertension or obesity that we know can lead to chronic illness and/or acute episodes. As surgeons, we may attend to an emergency appendectomy or traumatic injuries, or we may carry out a planned and pre-scheduled bariatric surgery for obesity. As rheumatologists, we may deal with recurring episodes of joint deterioration in arthritic patients, and have to judge when it's time for the patient to move to a different modality of care. We have to carefully evaluate and design our care pathways to fit the needs of the patient, not to accommodate the needs of the providers.

All of us may see patients who either adhere or don't to their treatment plan around drugs, therapies, and lifestyle recommendations. Historically we've seen adherence as beyond our control, and the responsibility of the patient. That's no longer the case. We have an obligation to discuss the reasons for non-compliance, and to try to find a treatment plan that achieves adherence. Some of our patients may want to combine our treatment with non-traditional medicine and/or nutritional approaches. We have expanded our services to include Eastern medicine and to put a strong focus on nutrition. Patient variation and individualism is growing, as are patient preferences for how they receive care.

Up until now, we've defined our responsibility rather narrowly and asked the patient to conform to the way we practice. It simply does not make sense that we would deal with all these patients using the same approaches. We need robust clinical approaches based on evidence and best practice. But our healthcare delivery processes, and our medical practices need to adapt to different contingencies, many of which cannot be predicted with certainty. Individualized care requires the coordination of the various elements of care so the patient truly is at the center.

One health system that is individualizing care while also engaging patients in that care is Minnesota's HealthPartners. By carefully assessing the health status of its members, it tailors a broad range of health and wellness offerings, including disease management programs, prevention, outreach, behavioral coaching, help lines, and computerized resources, in addition to individualized care pathways. HealthPartners also customizes its health and wellness offerings to address the culture and needs of the companies who purchase its plan.[19]

At SCPMG, physicians have helped develop approaches to ensure that our care fits the individual patient. For example, care managers reach out to patients with conditions such as osteoporosis, diabetes or hypertension to make sure they receive appropriate routine and preventive treatment from a variety of primary care and specialist physicians, pharmacists, nurses, dieticians, social workers, and lifestyle coaches. Through ongoing monitoring, treatment, education, and other support, we hope to slow disease progression and avoid flare-ups.

Personalized care is clearly seen in our approach to depression. Serious depression, including suicidal tendencies, is often very difficult to detect and monitor. We have put in place many approaches, including outreach, in-reach and online screenings, to reach those who are depressed. We monitor many of our at-risk patients, and have built quick response capabilities. While it remains difficult, these approaches can save lives. Recently a young man took our total health assessment at kp.org, our online patient portal. His answers to the assessment tripped a red flag for suicidal ideation, and his information was relayed to outreach. A care manager called the young man. He had indeed

Dr. Brian Nguyen, Physician Director of Clinical Strategic Goals Optimization

"There is a level of clinical care that is at the individual level—that goes to the uniqueness of patients. Good physicians do it naturally and others struggle. We need to focus on this. We've put systems in place, so much of the technical work of medicine is systematic and even automated. The next advance will be in the art of medicine. The topic of conversation has to change. We haven't done a good job around wellness. We don't have a good concept of it. For me, wellness is about how do patients live their lives? Do they live it happily? Do they enjoy what they do in their everyday life? It's not necessarily all about disease prevention. A large percent of what I see is stress related. We have to have this conversation with our patients and understand their drivers in life. It is an area that is uncomfortable for many physicians, but an area that patients are yearning for care in. There's a backlash from some patients who are dissatisfied with how medicine is practiced—and how drug driven, imaging driven and legally driven it is. They're looking for an alternative approach."

been contemplating suicide, and we set in place a number of measures that may have helped save his life.

Individualized care is also evident in the individually optimized care plan we develop for total joint recovery for each patient who has a knee replacement. Our regional chief of Orthopedic Surgery, Dr. Tad Funahashi, has led our physicians in the development of this approach, based in part on the assumption that patients' time is valuable, and that spending unneeded care in a hospital is not in their best interests. There is a predictable sequence of events after a knee replacement. In the past, we all thought we were efficiently helping our patients through this sequence. By looking at this from a patient's perspective, we realized how random and uncoordinated this seemed, and how much time was wasted. Most importantly, we realized that this slowed down the patient's recuperation. Funahashi and his team mapped out an efficient pathway that integrates the work of doctors, nurses, pharmacists, physical therapists, and others involved in post-operative care. The pathway is tailored to each post-surgical patient's condition, and the information is shared with the patient and family. Anxiety and uncertainty can be reduced if patients and families know what to expect and understand the care plan.

Take the Care to the Patient. Ironically for our profession, some of the most patient-centered things we can do for many patients will allow them to avoid office visits. We can provide them with access to tests and other information and self-service capabilities. Making greater use of virtual care and self-service can be a win-win. Patients don't want to spend unnecessary time making calls, visiting our offices, or waiting for call backs. It is becoming common to post test results on the kp.org website within hours of the test. This alleviates patient anxiety if the test is negative, and focuses our resources on getting back quickly and personally to those patients whose tests indicate a next step is needed.

Not surprisingly, the military is at the cutting edge of taking healthcare to the patient—in some of the most treacherous and dangerous of terrains. It has developed IT capabilities to connect these remote sites to the EMR and other healthcare information systems of the Military Healthcare System, and to provide battlefield decision support.[20] Closer to home, the Veteran's Health Administration has invested heavily in building Remote Patient Monitoring (RPM) into its chronic disease management processes. It uses the Health Hero Network's Health Buddy device. In its pilot demonstration of efficacy with congestive heart failure patients, use of the Health Buddy device for remote monitoring was associated with a 66 percent decrease in emergency department visits and a 60 percent decrease in hospital admissions.[21]

Because of the unprecedented explosion of computers and smartphones and the power of our EMR, we can now do many other care steps for patients without them having to come into a doctor's office. There is no reason to wait to order a routine test until the patient happens to show up for an appointment. Using automated phone calls, e-mail, or text messages, we can alert patients that it's time for the test and connect them to the website where they can easily make an appointment. An example of this is appropriate monitoring of patients on long-term medicines such as hypertensives who automatically have lab tests pended for electrolytes and renal functioning.

With home diagnostic capabilities and mobile health vans that can go to workplaces, we are beginning to truly respond to the busy lives of our many of our patients, and to the complicated demands placed upon frail patients or those with conditions that demand continual monitoring. For example, at-home blood pressure monitors securely upload the information to a patient's EMR and immediately report situations that are out of range and need a quick response. Patients in urgent need can then be directed to a same-day appointment with their physician, to a lab for follow-up testing, or for a very serious situation to the emergency room. With home monitoring, patients who are keeping their blood pressure under control may only need to come into the doctor's office once a year. What a relief for that patient! Our studies are showing that this type of care may be quite an effective way to keep blood pressure under control.[22] It provides real time response to indicators that may enable quick action to avert a medical crisis. It provides greater value to patients and society while consuming fewer resources.

Although virtual approaches may challenge some of our beliefs about how medicine should be practiced, we physicians need to explore their potential and learn how to best incorporate them into our daily practices. It's easier for us to have patients come to us—but it may not be easy for the patient. We may worry about the quality of these new approaches and about the virtual team that we now have to rely on. We may feel that systems that are being set up to avoid office visits are undermining our control, taking us out of the center, and even reducing our income. Yet the whole world is moving in a virtual direction. New communication vehicles and new technology create great opportunities to improve care and patient convenience while reducing costs. Rather than complain about how "medicine isn't what it used to be"—and it definitely isn't!—let's be part of figuring out how this can be a more fulfilling and impactful way for all of us to practice medicine.

Sharing Power—Healthcare is a Partnership with the Patient

Patient-focused care isn't just about making it more convenient or even pleasant for patients to do what we physicians think is best. It's about enabling patients to take responsibility for their health and empowering them to work with us to achieve the best possible outcomes *for them*. "What in the world are you talking about?" a doctor might say. "I'm the one who went through eight to ten years of training in order to know the best course of action." What is evidence-based practice all about if it isn't to enable us to tell the patient what needs to be done?

We know that much of what we prescribe for our patient has limited impact. The patient leaves our office and frequently does not follow the treatment plan. The reasons for not adhering to what we prescribe vary but often relate to a lack of time, money or convenience. Sometimes the patient does not understand our instructions or gets confused, particularly elderly patients. No matter how erudite we are and how careful we are in explaining, prescribing and treating, patients heal and recuperate in the context of their own lives.

In reality, patients do in many cases have a lot of information about their conditions even before they set foot in our examining rooms.[23] Just as important, more and more of our patients want to partner with their physician in determining courses of action. For them it may not be all about what is medically believed to be the best next step. They would like to weigh the odds in the context of their own values and life situation and make considered decisions. Is that really a bad thing? Not at all! In fact, partnering with the patient in making decisions may be the ultimate in patient-centric care.

Dr. Todd Sachs, Chief of Surgery for West Los Angeles

"Historically patients were more inclined to just listen to what you offered and say 'OK'. I love that patients are now coming in with data and asking lots of questions. It's more interactive. Information is more accessible and available to them, and in the comfort of their homes. For example, patients who come in with interest in bariatric surgery can have gone through a program where they learn the various options for weight control. If they choose the surgical route they know a lot about it. Patients who come with this kind of information have more questions. It's more enjoyable from a physician's standpoint. I can talk about the same thing over and over to different patients, but it's more enjoyable if we interact about it. I haven't found that it impacts the time I spend with a patient very much. Patients are often putting their life in my hands. You have to answer their questions and make sure they feel comfortable and build a relationship."

I believe partnering with patients makes our job both easier and more rewarding. I'm sure we've all had patients who were quite insistent on following what we feel to be an inferior or even dangerous course of action, and we definitely have a professional obligation to share our professional perspective and uphold our "do no harm" oath. Nevertheless, being patient-centered is very consistent with a focus on wellness. Patients who want to learn about their health and health conditions and play a role in deciding their own care should be encouraged.

Medical decisions are sometimes incredibly complicated, uncertain, and sensitive to various degrees of risk tolerance. Consider the over-diagnosis of prostate cancer with the use of the PSA screening test. Start with the fact that 60 percent of PSA-detected prostate cancers "would otherwise not go on to cause symptoms or death."[24] If a cancer is detected that may not ever manifest any health problems or symptoms, should it be treated? There are real possibilities for morbidity when treating prostate cancer, and potential side effects of surgery include incontinence and impotence. Should active surveillance be used instead?[25] How can a patient make sense of a cancer that exists but possibly should be left alone? This is a concept that is quite foreign to how Western culture has traditionally thought about cancer. It is an incredibly difficult situation. We physicians may have a point of view on how to treat this problem; in the end it is the patient who makes the decision on how to proceed. It's a good thing that many of our patients are oriented toward learning as much as they can, and toward being an active partner in medical decisions.

Being patient-centered is never more important than at the end of life. There is nothing that cries out more for respect and consideration and acting according to our patients' wishes than during the final stages of life. People should not have to give up their dignity and wishes just because they are near death or dying. Because we have the technology to keep people alive longer, we need to ensure we are using it in a manner consistent with the desires of the patient. This is why I think it's critical to have discussions with healthy patients to get them to start thinking about how they want their life to be at the end.

We should have total honesty with families and educate them about choices and uncertainties, while remaining cognizant of their personal beliefs and cultural milieu. Does a patient want hospice or palliative care, or prefer as aggressive a treatment as can be found? If a patient elects aggressive treatment, when does the patient think that enough is enough? I recommend that patients who are diagnosed with an advanced illness fill out a Physician Orders for Life-Sustaining Treatment (POLST) form.[26] This gives patients as explicit a voice as they want to have in their treatment options at the end of life.

Patients can help us co-design the care pathway that works best. They know what they value. They know the context of their lives, whereas we can only guess. Is the patient able to remember all the medications to take and all the foods to avoid? Am I prescribing medicine that the patient can afford? Is there a more cost-effective means that has a higher probability of compliance? Context is all important. Some patients can afford the co-payment and deductible, and others can't. That's not our job, say some physicians; it is the insurance company's problem. But of course it *is* our job to help patients improve their health status, and the patient's means is relevant to the course of action we prescribe.

Some patients have a great support system in their lives, composed of many family members and friends, whereas others are more alone. Some people need more support than others. Are we educating family members and bringing them into the decision making to the extent they can and want to be? Is our staff helping patients connect with support resources and following up to make sure they are not falling through the cracks? Being patient-centric demands that we worry about these things.

The Physician as Educator

Perhaps the most important thing that we as physicians can do for our patients is make sure that they are knowledgeable about how to take care of themselves and how to use healthcare resources to most effectively achieve their health goals. Education goes far beyond our conversations with patients and providing them with information sheets. We can connect patients to the resources that are available to help them work through their health challenges and to become more knowledgeable about general health issues and specific conditions they are facing.

We have increased our focus on health education at Kaiser Permanente. Doctors can refer patients to material on kp.org, or to in-person education and support groups dealing with nutrition and other lifestyle issues. We have programs on specific diseases and general health. In the area of diabetes, for example, there is a great deal of information on kp.org. This includes a list of diabetes self-management goals (such as controlling cholesterol, quitting smoking, and maintaining a healthy weight), information about typical prescription medications used with diabetes, and instructions on how to give oneself an insulin injection. KPSC also offers "HealthMedia Care for Diabetes" and "Emmi" online programs. HealthMedia Care is an interactive online quiz/consultation, the answers to which are used to create an individualized plan for management and control of the specific condition. It also includes additional links and resources, and triggers check-in e-mails and e-newsletters. Emmi offers online multimedia programs on such topics as checking blood sugar and using insulin. KPSC also offers its own diabetes videos on kp.org, along with a printable workbook to download. With these programs we are trying to engage our patients to actively take better care of themselves.

Of course, we also refer patients to the considerable resources outside of Kaiser Permanente. Many non-profits and government organizations offer a plethora of information and education on healthcare. Such well-known groups as the American Heart Association and the Centers for Disease Control offer consumer health information. The YMCA, the President's Council on Physical Fitness, and Project KaBOOM all offer resources and opportunities to encourage greater physical activity and physical fitness. The National Institutes of Health has downloadable publications and web pages about many health topics, such as depression, weight control, alcoholism, autism, and health concerns for travelers.

But we don't just give patients a list of resources. Our proactive healthcare team actively monitors their care and continually adjusts their care plans. We contact our patients to urge them to take advantage of the resources that will help them care for themselves, and we let them know about new resources. What can be more patient-centric than giving patients the knowledge to take responsibility for their health?

Although we physicians may not all practice medicine in a setting that provides us such rich support in making sure our patients are educated, we all need to find a way to connect patients to the many resources available in their communities and online. We are now able, as never before, to increase the impact of our care by enabling patients to better care for themselves. We can take heroic measures to diagnose and treat illness, but we need a team to achieve the best outcomes. And the patient is the most important member of that team!

Trend	Implications for Physicians	Am I effectively dealing with this trend now?
The Patient Experience		
	1. Patients are demanding high-quality experiences, not just high-quality care.	
Service Expectations		
	1. Organize around service to our patients, not just in ways that are convenient to us. 2. Increased emphasis on communication skills (the "bedside manner") and empathy	
Ease of Access and Use		
	1. Patients increasingly seek out healthcare services at places and times convenient for them—near their homes and at their places of work. 2. Physicians are reviewed and rated publicly/online.	
Cultural Sensitivity		
	1. Care is being delivered to an increasingly diverse population. 2. Language differences impede quality of care.	
Communication		
	1. Patients expect and need a written version of their diagnosis and prescriptions. 2. Ease of access to medical records will be an expected part of medical practice.	
Individualized Care		
	1. Culturally responsive and individualized care are two components of patient-centered care. 2. Patients expect various caregivers to create an integrated care pathway. 3. Effective care fits the context of patients' lives and beliefs.	
Reaching Out to Patients Proactively and Taking Care to Them		
	1. Aggressive, proactive care is essential to a preventive approach to medicine.	

Trend	Implications for Physicians	Am I effectively dealing with this trend now?
Patients as Partners		
	1. Many patients want to play an active role in their own healthcare. 2. Patients increasingly use electronic communication technologies to be active and educated partners in the care process. 3. The education of patients will be a much larger component of medicine. 4. Patients seek information from other sources.	

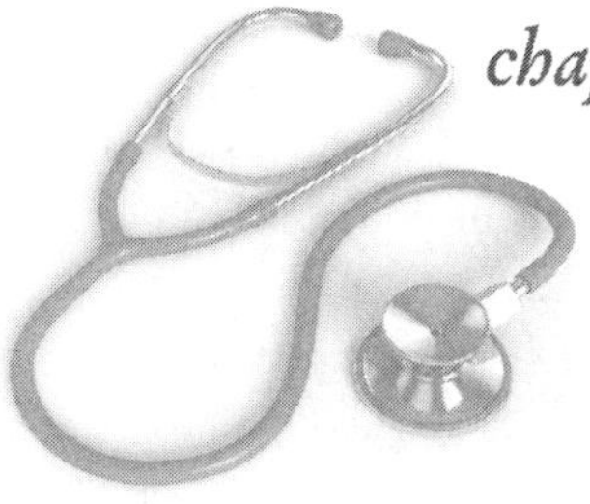

chapter four

Electronic Medical Records and Other IT Applications

We have all heard the term the "digital divide," usually in reference to particular segments in a society, like the more economically disadvantaged, who do not have access to computers and the Internet. In general, however, computers and the web permeate American society. Healthcare has been a laggard in this respect. The healthcare industry has been slow to embrace the potential of information technology to improve quality and increase value. But that is changing rapidly. The transition is rough, leading to a sea change in how we practice medicine. But the benefits for physicians and patients are great. It's inconceivable that physicians can continue to operate with storage rooms full of paper records and a model where patients must physically show up for every health problem. Failure to embrace technology will lead to catastrophic results in terms of cost, quality, access, and service.

You probably have some kind of computer or web-enabled device within reach of you right now, either in the guise of a smartphone, a tablet computer, or an actual laptop or desktop. But in the US, only 69 percent of primary care physicians use an EMR. The situation is vastly different in such countries as New Zealand, Norway, and the Netherlands, where the figure is over 95 percent.[1] Despite committing a much higher percentage of our GDP to healthcare, the US does not have the healthiest population, and one reason may be our slowness in taking advantage of IT technology to improve quality and reduce cost.

The American Medical Association in 2006 enumerated the many benefits of using an EMR, including the integration of patient care, reduction in medical errors, increased coordination and efficiency of healthcare delivery, and reduced transaction costs.[2] So why is the profession of medicine in the US one of the victims of the digital divide? One major barrier has been cost. The myriad of healthcare systems and medical practices around the country have each had to shoulder the cost of developing and/or purchasing, tailoring, and implementing an EMR system. For many, this has been prohibitive. Yet even when systems have been able to make this investment, up to 30 percent fail and others encounter far more difficulties than expected.[3]

An often cited reason for the slow uptake has been reluctance by physicians to change the way we practice medicine. Trinity Health, the large US Catholic healthcare provider, invested over $400 million over a decade in its EMR that is used by its forty-four hospitals and eight thousand physicians. CEO Joe Swedish is quoted as saying, "It started out as a massive technology project with a clinical change component" but turned into "a massive clinical and cultural change project, with a technology foundation."[4]

Even in countries where a national health system has mandated and guided the transition to EMRs, the pathway to that goal has not been smooth or quick. The change process in Denmark, a country that was an early EMR adopter, has taken twenty years, and there are still Danish hospitals that are not fully on the system.[5] In order to enable greater local capability to adapt the national EMR system more fully to local needs and practice patterns, the British National Health System has recently abandoned its centralized approach and has given increased choice of vendors and systems to local hospitals. The image has moved from one large monolithic system to connected systems around the country.[6]

Early introductions of EMR systems are often accompanied by frustration and even resistance as generic systems that don't completely fit our work are stuck in place and skeptical physicians quickly learn that off-the-shelf systems make it harder, not easier, to do our work.[7] A good example is my neighboring system, Cedars-Sinai, one of the finest and most technologically advanced systems in the country. In 2002 the medical center spent $34 million on an order entry system for medications, labs, and procedures, only to withdraw it amid physician outrage about its complexity (and constraints), the amount of time it took to use it, and its lack of flexibility.[8]

Indeed, my own system, Kaiser Permanente, experienced many similar challenges during our initial implementation—and our physicians were understandably upset by its time demands, the overload of information, the long training hours that were required, and associated loss of productivity and excessive workload. That was a very difficult time for all of us. We're still working through refining our workflows and workloads. We had learned through earlier IT implementations that for this transition to be effective, physicians would have to adjust to the software while it was being fine-tuned to adjust to the physician's practice. Fortunately there are many visionary physicians in SCPMG who believed that we could make electronic records and IT work for us. These physicians have been steadily building the systems to address the needs of our members and improve their health.

Dr. Brian Nguyen, Physician Director of Clinical Strategic Goals Optimization

"My first two years at KP we had paper charts and now it's all electronic. I love it. A younger physician who sees new electronics expects there to be bugs and data problems. New smartphones, for example, have bugs and they get worked out. We're used to that process. It's a different approach to technology—get it and start using it instead of always wanting a perfect product from the beginning. Technology improves as we use it and find the bugs and change things. Young physicians embraced that concept. Things are so much more efficient now compared to the paper chart days."

HealthConnect™ (KP's EMR system) and our Permanente Online Interactive Network Tool (POINT) system, which integrates our many component systems and enables the management of the care of a panel of patients, have been integral to our progress toward our goals. IT capability has been a key enabler of prevention, has helped us tailor care to individuals, and has improved our value ratio of outcomes to cost. Our physicians and other providers now have access to timely and complete information to inform their decision making, and this has enabled us to fully utilize the skills and capabilities of our physicians and staff to increase the value that we deliver.

It isn't enough simply to create digital records where they used to be paper records. Electronic medical records should not be a fancy filing system. The IT systems are information platforms that allow each of us to be more effective, and more importantly, they allow the whole team to effectively communicate and work together to improve care. The real breakthroughs, though, have been in the innovative ideas from our physician leaders about how to work differently to be more effective.

The Shift is Inevitable, and It's About Time

The US has been slow in adopting EMRs, but that's changing. The federal government has passed three acts since 2009 promoting electronic health/medical records:

- Children's Health Insurance Program (CHIP) Reauthorization Act
- Health Information Technology for Economic and Clinical Health (HITECH) Act (part of the 2009 American Recovery and Reinvestment Act—ARRA)
- 2010 Affordable Care Act (ACA)

The HITECH Act of 2009 is notable for its incentive programs: It offers an estimated $27 billion dollars for Medicare and Medicaid incentive payments to eligible providers that make the switch to electronic records. Requirements for the payments include demonstrating that the electronic records are used meaningfully for such things as electronic prescribing, that the information contained in the records can be exchanged among necessary health professionals for care coordination, and that the information can be reported to national bodies to compile clinical quality and other measures.[9] Significantly, HITECH will eventually penalize physicians who do not adopt EMRs. The penalties include decreasing Medicare/Medicaid reimbursements for doctors who haven't adopted certified EMRs by 2015.[10]

Given this sweep of recent legislation, the train has left the station. Regardless of the ultimate shape of healthcare reform, the use of EMRs will be integral to the way we all practice medicine. Some doctors may be early adopters of technology and some may be much more traditional and slow to change. Younger doctors who have grown up with the rise of computers in society are having an easier time adopting EMR technology in their practices than some of us older physicians, who may have had to learn to type! However, I have seen in my system that even the doctors who have been dragged practically kicking and screaming to the EMR experience the benefits. They appreciate having patient information at their fingertips that enables them to know their patient's history and do a better job of providing care.

Dr. Todd Sachs, Chief of Surgery for West Los Angeles

"EMR took us further toward our goal of prevention and patient oriented care. It was one of the toughest changes for us. It required a change in the culture. No one would ever give it up now. EMR enhances our quality. And it makes patients feel so much better about the care they receive. When patients came in twenty-six years ago I would say 'I'm so sorry I don't have the chart.' Now it's 'let's sit down together and see what your tests show.' I can show her the x-rays, go through it, discuss the doctor's interpretations, and see lab results in seconds. It's improved service and it's the proper type of care to give someone."

I remember the "good old days" when the chart was sometimes not there when you needed it—lost in the slow bureaucracy of the system or misplaced in a stack of unfiled documents. The chart might have been incomplete, missing x-rays, test results, or records. And we did not have access to patients' charts when they were being seen by other clinicians. We could see only fragments of a patient's history and concurrent conditions. We doctors developed all kinds of coping strategies to deal with these constraints, but they also limited the knowledge we had about a patient to deliver the best possible care. Besides getting lost, paper records are vulnerable to the environment they're stored in and the kind of paper they're written on. After Hurricane Katrina hit in 2005, one million people in New Orleans lost their medical records.[11]

Consider this: why can we use our smartphones to access our bank accounts, pay all our bills online, order practically anything from vendors across the globe via the web, and even see our entire credit histories online, but still have to thumb through an ancient file folder that is most likely an incomplete record of a patient's health history? Put yourself in your patients' shoes: why can't they see their complete medical record online? It is, after all, their lives and health. What a boon to have it as conveniently accessible as possible. Partnerships have emerged between healthcare providers like the Cleveland Clinic, Mayo Clinic, Kaiser Permanente and New York-Presbyterian to work with technology firms such as Microsoft and Google to address technical issues involved in transferring medical records to personal health records that are easy to use.[12] In the future, people's medical records will be available via their mobile device—this is already happening in our system.

Integrating Care Delivery

EMRs in their most basic form are simply electronic versions of a patient's record. It's how the data get used that determines whether it promotes higher quality and more efficient healthcare or are simply a new (and perhaps more time consuming) way of recording information. For example, having a common system on a common platform enables multiple physicians and other members of the care team to enter, access, and share information about the same patient with each other. Having a completely electronic medical record will play a large role in knitting together the profoundly and distressingly fragmented contemporary healthcare system. EMRs can enable truly interconnected, effective, holistic care—helping to monitor care, providing alerts, and shouldering some of the load of care coordination, order entry, and administrative documentation. No more subjecting patients to yet another blood test or x-ray because we can't access the one that was done last week in another office or during an emergency room visit. And because we can reconcile all the medications that a patient is taking and provide patients with clear reports of what drugs they should currently be taking, we should see far fewer instances of patients being readmitted to the hospital because they had a prescription changed during a former stay, but after going home to a whole bag of the old meds, ended up taking the wrong ones.

This systematization and record sharing enables healthcare team members in other locations to have access to information that used to require a physician to page through and pull information from a paper file. Others can check to make sure that when the patient shows up for an exam, the blood test has already been done and the results are posted. Used wisely, this virtual capability frees doctors up to do what we do best: interact with, diagnose, and treat our patients.[13]

HealthConnect coordinates and integrates care between primary care physicians, specialty care, the pharmacy, the lab, and radiology—and makes records available to all the staff who care for the patient. The base of our EMR is a system from Epic, a company that makes software for large and medium-sized healthcare entities. To improve the functionality of our IT systems, we have our own version of a Skunk Works (MDs, PhDs, informaticists, programmers, developers, linguists, and others), who collaborate with our physicians and work on enhancements.

As seen in Figure 1, we now have in place a complex system with fifteen separate modules that communicate with the HealthConnect software. I know that it helps doctors make better medical decisions. Dr. Julia Bae, the medical director of the Kern County Medical Center and previously the asthma champion for the medical center, noted how the EMR system helps improve the overall care of asthma patients: "I could pull up detailed medical information on every asthma patient in my medical center including when they picked up their rescue inhalers and preventive medications. This allowed me to reach out to the patients who are at risk and improve their overall asthma management."

For SCPMG, implementation was not easy. Beyond the mechanics of using the system, we had to change how we work. Physicians experienced increasing pressure managing a continuous flow of data in their in-baskets. We developed and conducted a series of training programs to educate physicians and staff in the new systems. We developed shortcuts (smart phrases) to facilitate data entry. Perhaps most importantly, we redesigned workflows to optimize team work.

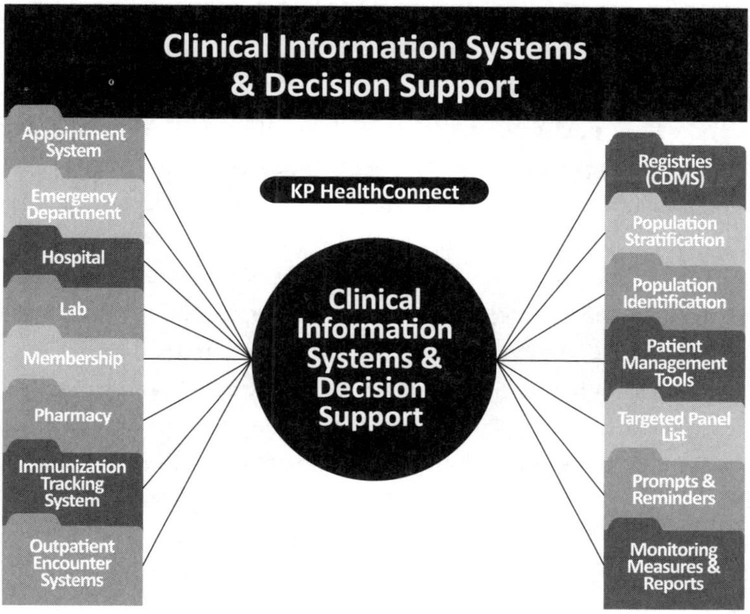

Figure 1: *KP's Electronic Medical System*

Workflow Enhancement: Physicians Doing Physicians' Work

As every industry adopting new technology has discovered, you can't take advantage of new capabilities and do work the old way. The EMR is much more than just the translation of paper records onto digital records. Its real power comes from algorithms and applications that enable more effective information sharing and care management. If we don't change the way the healthcare team works, physicians can be overwhelmed by all the new capabilities and responsibilities—not to mention by the increased speed and complexity when patients are able to access their own records and initiate their own care. The right information technology can help us greatly improve quality by increasing prevention, reducing safety risks, taking a disease life cycle approach, and creating individualized patient care paths, but only if we work as a team.

Working with our hospital systems, our clinic administrators, and other team members, we at SCPMG built tools that take work (particularly transactional work) off the plate of our physicians and move it into newly defined roles for each member of the care team. We enhanced the contribution and responsibilities of every team member so that every point of contact with the patient enhances personalized care delivery. On the EMR, members of the team see a screen tailored to their role in the system of care. For example, receptionists in physician offices see a list of all scheduled patients, and it tells where the care gaps are. So when a patient shows up for an appointment, the receptionist can say, "I see you haven't had your mammogram. Let's make an appointment."

The multiple physicians and other members of the team who see the same diabetic patient are connected by the electronic health record and have collective responsibility for fulfilling all of the patient's medical needs. Specific tasks are distributed to different team members, based on their skills and expertise, creating a virtual team of caregivers. For example, pharmacy aides and pharmacists are responsible for managing phone calls concerning drug refills, side effects and dosing. While team members don't have the same skills, all are alerted and can recognize when there is a gap or a problem. When a patient presents with diabetes that is out of control, for example, team members can recognize the problem and direct the patient to get needed care.

Decision Support

An integrated EMR also provides a platform for physician decision support. Busy doctors face a world where knowledge is growing exponentially, patients expect personalized care, and physicians have to assure quality and use resources wisely to deliver high value. That's a lot to think about and remember. We physicians should not have our decisions constrained by a system, but we appreciate having alerts, best practice advice, and knowledge about the latest research readily available to help us to make better decisions.

Under the leadership of Dr. Paul Minardi, our medical director of Operations, a group of thoughtful physicians working with pharmacy, radiology and analytical support have built first-order decision support into our HealthConnect system. They have considered hundreds of ideas from our physicians and determined priorities where decision support would be the most valuable. Hard- and soft-stop safety alerts advise doctors if they have prescribed a drug that has adverse interactions with other drugs that the patient is taking—or if the patient has risk factors that are associated with adverse impact. Best practice information is provided, along with information about generics that have been found to be as efficacious and consequently a better value than a brand name drug.

Building decision support into the EMR helps us avoid critical errors. We may lose track of how much of a drug has been prescribed and not realize we're approaching the safety limit. Or, we may not know that the patient hasn't filled his prescription, and that lack of adherence underlies our inability to help him get his blood pressure under control. We may need to be able to refer to the latest FDA guidance in talking with a patient who makes inappropriate drug requests based on pharmaceutical advertisements. Whether as memory aids or information sources, decision support is reassuring to highly knowledgeable but very busy professionals. Ironically, a peril in the use of automated ordering systems that are part of EMR systems is that it's too easy to click on the wrong box and order the wrong drug or test. So it's consoling to know that there are safety checks to alert us if we make a choice that carries safety risks. The decision about what to prescribe or what action to take lies with the physician, but the information and alerts are there as aids.

"Our vision is to have countless safety nets running in the background—spinning 24/7 searching out patient needs and ensuring execution."

– Dr. Paul Minardi, SCPMG Regional Medical Director of Operations

We have also tied first-order decision support to our registries, so that those with chronic conditions such as diabetes are automatically evaluated at every visit, in fact, whether they come in or not. Their care gaps, preventive treatment, and treatment needs are identified. This provides support to our physicians in managing their patient panels. In the area of diabetes, in one cohort of 10,410 patients, this capability was associated with increases in LDL and A1c testing, and a decrease in both indicators. Our complete care approach was associated with an increase in participation in health education programs of 42.5 percent for this cohort (see Table 1).

Increased Rates of Testing	
increase in LDL testing	7.1%
increase in A1c testing	5.5%
Better Scores	
decreased average A1c	.55
decreased average LDL	6.32
increased % Hbg A1c <8	28.7%
increased % LDL <100	7%
Greater Participation in Health Education	
increased % participation in health education programs	42.5%

Figure 2: *Diabetes Complete Care Results (Data from cohort group of 10,410 patients followed for a twelve month period beginning January 2010.)*

Dr. Minardi's vision is "to have countless safety nets running in the background—spinning 24/7 searching out patient needs and ensuring execution." Many of the things that are noticed are transactional—informed by the patient's needs but not requiring judgment by the physician. Physicians can rely on the virtual team to identify the need and initiate care steps.

Get Ready: We're in the Midst of a Sea Change in Dealing with Patients

The EMR doesn't decrease the importance of clinical judgment, nor does it substitute for the caring and discerning relationship of the physician with the patient. During an office visit or in the hospital room, we need to make sure that we don't ignore our patient and only focus on the computer screen. Making sure the EMR documentation is correct doesn't trump a doctor's responsibility to provide a compassionate bedside manner. Yet incorporating IT capabilities into our practices is part of a revolution throughout our society that has inevitably changed the nature of service delivery and established a different set of expectations and behavior of both service providers and service purchasers.

We no longer expect to have to stand in line to see a teller to do banking. We can move money around—even large sums of money, pay bills, and do a variety of banking tasks from the convenience of our home. We can research information on the Internet to assist us on financial matters. We don't want to have to go through a broker to invest our money, although we may want to talk to a financial adviser when we're making important financial decisions. We want to be empowered with information and convenient service that's responsive to our individual needs. And we physicians have to understand that that's just what our patients want in their healthcare.

Empowering Patients. We all know that many of our patients are already taking steps to empower themselves. They are reading and learning more about health and aggressively pursuing online resources to learn about prevention and health conditions that affect them, their loved ones and friends. They are pursuing multiple opinions, and in some cases looking at alternative healthcare options such as acupuncture or natural medicines. Aggressive self-management by patients is a good thing. It frequently leads to greater adherence to healthy and health-restoring regimens, and makes it easier to have a problem-solving discussion with the patient, and to work together in making tough treatment decisions. And yes, it also stretches our skills and energies to deal with such engaged patients. Yet the opposite is worse. How often do we bemoan the lack of adherence that leads to pre-diabetics becoming diabetic too young, or to controllable hypertension leading to a possibly preventable stroke?

The use of modern IT capabilities is integral to empowering patients and to making healthcare more convenient. In keeping with our belief that prevention underpins high-quality healthcare, we at SCPMG are using new communication media to ensure that our patients take all necessary preventive steps, and that they know enough about their disease to alter their behavior to speed recovery, prevent complications, and slow down progression.

Kp.org allows enormous direct, secure, and protected communication to and from patients. Our patients go there for electronic access to most of their test results—most within hours after the test. They also can access a variety of other personal health information, including a list of their allergies, immunizations, health conditions, healthcare reminders, patient instructions, recent lab or x-ray results, a current health summary, and a health risk questionnaire. Having everything in writing and available to patients online at all times helps them with ongoing care self-management.[14]

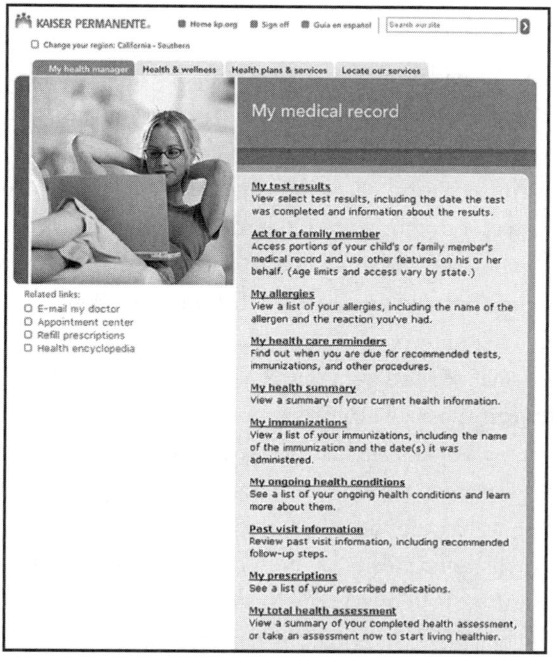

Figure 3: *kp.org patient medical record web page*

Kp.org also enables self-service through features such as ordering prescription refills, scheduling appointments, and requesting referrals online.[15] Patients also can send secure e-mails to their doctors, nurses, or pharmacists. In addition, patients are able to get medical advice from a clinician or arrange same day or next day appointments as needed.

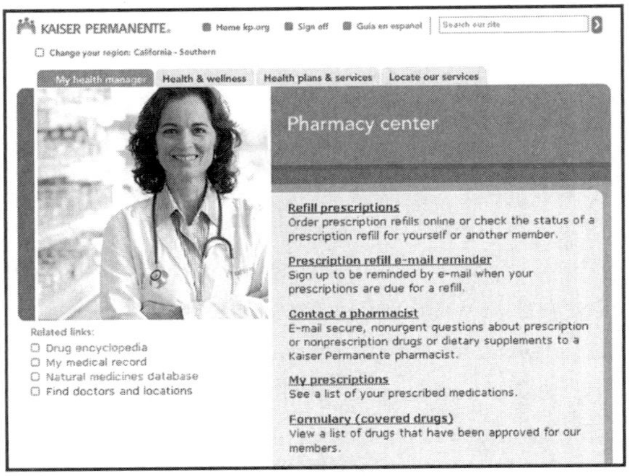

Figure 4: *kp.org pharmacy access web page for patients*

Kp.org maintains a vast amount of health information available twenty-four/seven. This provides our physicians with one more tool to help patients manage their health. Our patients can access general information about wellness, various health conditions, diseases and medications. In addition, they can find basic information about our medical centers and other facilities, whether a particular doctor speaks a particular language, and take a virtual visit to the hospital unit they will be visiting. Also available on this website are health risk assessments, and educational programs. For example, any interested patient can take an online program on reducing stress, which includes a survey to create a personalized program for managing stress and reducing its symptoms. Patients can also access information about face-to-face classes and support groups in the system, such as breast and colon cancer support groups, an infant CPR class, and a menopause class. All of this is readily searchable without calling or visiting the office, and at the convenience of the patient.

We also use IT to help us reach out to our members about issues important to their health. If you're in our system, HealthConnect may trigger a prerecorded robocall, or an e-mail or text message (whichever you prefer) if you have not received a needed flu shot. The reminder is a friendly and polite way to educate our patients and, frankly, to nag them a little into doing what is in their best interest. We also reach out to our members about public health emergencies. For example, during the Station wildfire in the San Gabriel Mountains in 2009, we were able to quickly inform all of our members in affected areas about the dangers posed by the smoke, and to give them guidance about their levels of risk. We also provided information on how to care for themselves and their families. Because our registries are connected to our EMR, we're able to reach out to affected patients when the FDA issues guidance about a drug that they are taking, and provide them with information about how to work with their physician to determine their best course of action.

Bringing Healthcare to the Patient. Healthcare has historically not been a very convenient service for patients, who have had to leave work, drive to the doctor's office, wait their turn, and then get sent from office to office for tests, consults, and follow-ups. Patients often hand carried test results and records and made calls to different offices to try and coordinate their care. In the meantime, we physicians sat in our own offices, tending our business, leaving patients to fend for themselves. And generally, we worried about our patients who came to see us, not the ones who didn't.

Now through technology and IT-enabled approaches such as home monitoring and mobile services, and by providing healthcare in employer sites and shopping centers, we can reach out to our patients without them needing to come into the office. These remote delivery systems can be completely linked into the EMR. Home self-monitoring and self-care delivery is the next frontier, and we're approaching it quickly.

Just as it is now possible to provide electronic decision support for physicians, we can do the same for patients. This will better enable them to take care of themselves on a daily basis. Their medical testing and treatment courses of events can be built into their calendars, so that they are alerted when it's time for medication, which is a great support for the frail or forgetful elderly, or the busy and preoccupied citizen at large. We are exploring the value of providing hand-held devices for patients who have been released from the hospital to remind them of the regimen that has been prescribed. This will reduce the frequency in which they come into the emergency room because they've not adhered to important orders that would have kept them stable and/or promoted healing. We're experimenting with virtual visits, because we know the criticality of making follow-up contact to ensure that patients understand their orders and/or to enable visual contact to examine whether healing is happening as anticipated. We are also exploring teledermatology.

Virtual capabilities especially hold promise for monitoring and even treating chronically ill patients. For example, we are exploring the use of in-home dialysis machines that concurrently give biophysical profiles of the patient that can be downloaded into their EMR. We anticipate that soon we'll have reliable algorithms that will analyze the data and alert the case manager and the patient when there is a problem that needs attention.

Building on the capabilities afforded by the EMR, the use of secure e-mails for doctor/patient communication represents a huge step forward in providing quality medical care and addressing issues of convenience for the patient. For example, our studies show that among patients with diabetes and hypertension, the use of secure e-mails is associated with an increase in the quality of care as measured by HEDIS, and an improvement in glycemic (HbA1c), cholesterol, and blood pressure screening and control.[16]

Healthcare has only begun to scratch the surface of what is possible through virtual care. We need to investigate when virtual care makes sense and when higher-touch, interpersonal interaction is preferable. While I support the adoption of new technology, we must guard against carrying this too far. An in-person, hands-on physical examination is still the critical capability in a physician's toolkit—and in many cases sufficient to yield a reliable diagnosis. Our profession has already gravitated too far, in my opinion, toward over-utilizing fancy tests and equipment, and virtual care will further reduce hands-on, eyeball-to-eyeball interaction. Yet it also offers huge promise if used appropriately.

We definitely have to learn when it makes sense to do things virtually, and conveniently, versus when it is more important to the well-being of the patient to make personal face-to-face contact. At the same time, we have to acknowledge that our current approaches are costly in terms of everyone's time and other resources. And, we have to acknowledge that healthcare will not escape the implications of the new service expectations and changing modalities of communication that characterize our societies.

There is an inexorable pull toward using technology for routine tasks, to increase reliability and automaticity of communications, to connect with patients in ways they prefer, and to make our scarce healthcare resources go further. I'm certain that many of us are wondering what the reimbursement approach is that will accompany this transition—and whether healthcare will become a commodity. Indeed, there is extreme pressure for the more routine parts of healthcare to be carried out as cost effectively as possible, and that means change for us all.

If we redesign the workflow well, the use of new technologies offers us the possibility to spend our time where we can add the most value. As we learn to better understand the costs, benefits and limitations of these technologies, and to stratify our patients in terms of risk and their preferred mode of care, we should improve the positive outcomes for the entire healthcare system. Approaches to reimbursement that rely on outcomes should create a win-win situation by rewarding the outcomes regardless of the means by which the care is delivered. But these positive outcomes will only happen if we physicians are part of crafting the solutions, not resistors who ultimately are the victims of others' solutions.

Knowledge Generation

Frankly, an EMR used mindfully is an awesome tool, both for care delivery and for increasing our fundamental knowledge about healthcare. In addition to being a boon on a patient-by-patient basis, its search capabilities enable us to populate clinical trials more quickly than through traditional means.[17] It also provides a database that can be mined for rigorous comparative effectiveness research, appropriately protecting the privacy of all patient information. Comparative healthcare effectiveness research is a trend that is growing as we realize what can be done with the wealth of data in our electronic systems.[18] The legal requirement that all new EMRs coming online in the next few years be interoperable will only serve to increase the body of data able to be mined and analyzed to generate a greater understanding of the efficacy of our approaches.

Already the ability to mine the data of our more than eight million records across all of KP nationally gives us a huge and very diverse population to extract information about treatments, medicines and outcomes. We can easily measure the degree to which our outreach programs are working. We have the ability to very quickly address issues like "Does this treatment work for the elderly, or for children?"—questions that are rarely addressed during clinical trials.

We have over 120,000 total joint replacements in our KP inter-regional registry, which allows us to look at multiple variables from medical center-specific issues to the nature of the implant, the procedure, and specific technique.

Over the past three to four years, under the leadership of our regional chief of Orthopedic Surgery, Dr. Tad Funahashi, we have been working as a part of the International Consortium of Orthopaedic Registries (ICOR) collaborative, which is sponsored by the FDA, in connecting all the orthopedics registries from across the world. This collaboration yields over two million registered joints, allowing the quick surfacing of bogus or misleading claims from vendors and the identification of underperforming devices. Recently, one company introduced a gender-specific knee replacement, but through the patterns in our registry our physicians found that there was no real difference in performance. Analysis of data from Australian registries in the collaboration have shown that almost all of the new technologies that have been introduced in the past several years are underperforming established joint replacements although the new technologies cost more.

The Power of Numbers: Total Joint Replacements in Our Registries, 2011

KP Inter-Regional Registry:
Over 120,000 total joint replacements

ICOR Collaborative (combined worldwide joint registries, sponsored by the FDA):
Over 2 million total joint replacements

This many knee replacements let us identify bogus or misleading claims from manufacturers and identify underperforming devices, and understand the comparative effectiveness of various devices in different populations of patients.

Such comparative effectiveness research supplements traditional clinical trials. Although randomized trials are the gold standard, comparative effectiveness research is often as compelling to physicians because it investigates how the treatment works in actual practice. Clinical trials enroll people who are younger, healthier and more drug compliant than a typical "real world" population, and there is some controversy over whether clinical trial results can easily be successfully translated into real world results.[19] Clinical effectiveness research doesn't have this problem.

As EMRs become more compatible and interoperable, our work as physicians will increasingly contribute not only to improving the health of our own patients, but also to establishing databases that will allow a systematic review and improvement of the drugs, devices, and treatments that we use. It may make us squirm, as we realize that we may be using approaches discovered to be ineffective or that there are effective alternatives that are less costly. Yet, our integrity as a profession depends on continually shining a light on our practice and ensuring that we are indeed delivering safe and efficacious care. Most important, this means that our profession will be leading the way in achieving high-value healthcare with outcomes that instill pride in all of us.

Dealing with Overload

New technologies hold great promise. A diabetic can be part of a virtual community that includes blogs and questions and answers from doctors, pharmacists, care managers, and other patients, and that includes links to many resources, including announcements of face-to-face support groups. A patient can send in a photo of a rash to a dermatologist to see if an appointment is needed, thus potentially avoiding an unnecessary trip to the doctor's office. Through home monitoring after release from the hospital, patients with congestive heart failure tend to need significantly fewer home nursing visits while at the same time reporting increased quality of life.[20]

We're just beginning to learn what is possible and desirable, and what these new capabilities mean for physicians, other healthcare providers, patients, payers, and families. How do we leverage things like Twitter, Facebook and the iPhone? How much face-to-face interaction is needed for patients with different risk factors, technological capabilities, and personal care knowledge? What are the new outreach obligations for physicians who can now scan their patients' EMRs to discover which patients need notification of new FDA guidance about their drugs? What are our responsibilities to patients who do not come in for care?

The implementation of KP HealthConnect was a transformational event for SCPMG physicians. It permitted easy access to the entire medical record, improved communication between healthcare teams and our members and permitted tremendous gains in quality. But there were substantial challenges as well. At the time of implementation only about 40 percent of our physicians were proficient typists and computer skills were lacking amongst many senior physicians. Early in the deployment, we had not yet designed our new workflows, and many of the clerical tasks that would come to be performed by support staff were being done by physicians on top of all their other tasks.

As a result, many physicians had to work numerous hours in the evening and weekends to complete tasks in the electronic in-basket. To address this challenge a multispecialty team of physicians (led by family physician Mark Eastman, MD, of Riverside) developed a program called Pathway to Proficiency. It was designed to be taught by fellow physicians to develop the skills required to be proficient in the new electronic medical record era. In 2009 the program trained nearly 200 physicians in three sessions at an offsite location away from demands of the medical office. According to Dr. Eastman:

The outcome was far from certain as this group of struggling physicians convened on the first day. There was a mood of discouragement amongst many of the attendees because of their inability to keep up with the work load. But by the afternoon of the first day there was a dramatic change in the mood. The elbow-to-elbow support provided by the physician trainers gave the attendees a real sense that "I can do this!"

Each evening we had a computer lab with physician trainers in attendance. And despite a Lakers playoff game and an American Idol finale, about 80 percent of the physicians attended the evening computer labs, some staying as late as one o'clock in the morning. It was both exhausting and exhilarating for the physician trainers. We knew we were making a lasting difference in the lives of these physicians.

On the last day, as the attendees streamed out, some of them had tears in their eyes as they thanked us for our efforts. Many said that the Pathway to Proficiency seminar "saved my career." Some said, "It was the best use of educational time I have ever experienced."

But one physician's reaction stands out in my mind. An endocrinologist approached me. As he shook my hand he said, "Before this seminar I was planning to leave Kaiser Permanente. Now I'm going to stay. You saved my career."

We were overwhelmed with these expressions of gratitude and understood that this was something that needed to continue for years to come.

Pathway to Proficiency has been adopted by numerous KP regions around the nation and is now taught at the local KP medical centers to hundreds of physicians every year.

Taking full advantage of the new IT capabilities puts new pressures on already busy physicians. Dr. Brian Nguyen points out that the EMR enables the management of care and outcomes of an entire panel of patients, not just patient by patient. For example, a physician can look across the panel of two thousand patients and identify patterns and progress across the diabetics in the panel. This leads to the ability to identify and reach out to those who have care gaps or whose indicators are moving in the wrong direction. The record readily tells the physician who needs what care. Results from tests come back more quickly, enabling much quicker decisions about the next care steps. But, according to Nguyen, "We have to change with these new capabilities and increased speed. In the past there were delays. Now more is compressed in a shorter timeframe. What used to be done across several visits is now done in a single one. The psychological stress is higher. Physicians need more resources to deal with this."

As we physicians have become more proficient with the EMR, and as new capabilities have been added to the system, we rely on it more and more. The implementation of an EMR puts more burden on the physician —to enter and review information, to communicate, and to respond quickly. Using electronic communications to detect unmet needs and to reach out to and respond to patients represents a new demand on physician time, albeit one that cannot be accounted for in terms of numbers of scheduled office visits. This is why we involve the entire healthcare team in a workflow that takes many routine tasks off the plate of the physician. Doctors don't have to have their fingers on every little aspect of patients' care. The benefit comes when the system is enhanced and becomes a tool for physicians rather than an administrative obligation.

We know that this system isn't perfect, and we continue to introduce elements to improve it. The demand on our healthcare system is growing while resources are not. For that reason, we all need to work to make this transition successful, and to enable the many innovations that will be required to derive full advantage.

Electronic in-box overload is not only an issue for doctors–it's rampant throughout Western society. We physicians need to learn how to deal with the information deluge, since we can't ignore it! We need to learn to effectively and efficiently use modern information technology to make us better informed and able to deliver more proactive and integrated care to our patients. We need to lead the development of the new healthcare systems that incorporate these approaches in a manner that doesn't overwhelm us. In today's world, where information tools make possible great leaps in exchange and application of knowledge, enhanced communication, and aids to memory and decision making, it's simply inconceivable that our profession can continue to operate without wholeheartedly embracing new technology.

Trend	Implications for Physicians	Am I effectively dealing with this trend now?
Integrated & Complete Care		
	1. The physician is only one of many contributing relevant information to the record. 2. We're part of a defacto virtual team dealing with the patient, a team held together by common information about the patient and interdependent care pathways.	
Virtual Care		
	1. Our work will increasingly be prescribed by well-specified care pathways and standard processes, and often virtual connections between caregivers. 2. Adherence to IT system requirements and processes provide a basis for coordination. 3. More use of electronic media in communicating with patients	
Transparency		
	1. All care steps are open to scrutiny. 2. Mistakes can't be buried. We must learn from them.	
Knowledge Generation & Comparative Effectiveness Research (stemming from EMR-based databases)		
	1. We'll be part of an ongoing research community by virtue of contributing to registries and other databases. 2. Steady stream of new knowledge requires continual adjustment of practice patterns. 3. A community of practice provides support for learning. 4. Decision support will be built into the EMR.	
Continual IT-Enabled Advances in Care Delivery Approaches and Processes		
	1. Continual incorporation of new applications and associated work process changes. 2. Patients have new expectations for communication.	

Trend	Implications for Physicians	Am I effectively dealing with this trend now?
Patient Information, Education, Empowerment		
	1. Increased modalities for patient education; physician and staff responsible to connect patient to useful resources. 2. Health educators are part of the team. 3. Educated patients are more active in questioning care prescriptions. 4. Patients expect timely feedback and responsiveness.	
Overload		
	1. Learn to rely on and trust the team. 2. Develop new habits to deal with complex communication streams.	

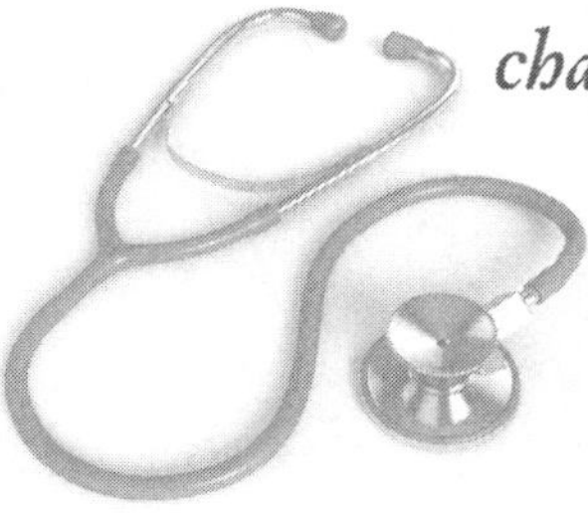

chapter five

Goals, Measurement and Accountability

Great healthcare systems, like other great organizations, lead based on performance. For this, you need discipline, focus, and accountability, to drive for results. I have been dead set on turning SCPMG into a great physician partnership whose care is among the best in the world. In doing this I have relied on measurements, accountability, and quality performance incentives.*

Society has been moving steadily toward increased measurement of healthcare with a focus on outcomes. We are being measured by a whole host of external groups.[1] With the advent of reimbursement for outcomes, measurement will lie at the heart of the resource flow for the entire healthcare system. We'll be accountable whether we like it or not. Less emphasis will be placed on pay for volume of activity, and more on the actual value of the care that is delivered to individuals and society. It has already started. For example, the US health insurer WellPoint will no longer give payment increases to hospitals if they don't score high enough on a treatment quality index.[2]

* *The Kaiser Foundation Health Plans and Kaiser Foundation Hospitals have no part in determining the incentives that SCPMG creates for physicians.*

Some Groups and Organizations that Measure Healthcare Providers, Plans and Hospitals in the US

HEDIS

- "Healthcare Effectiveness Data and Information Set." US health plan performance measures. Seventy-five measures over eight care "domains."[3]

Joint Commission Core Measures

- Hospital inpatient quality measures.[4]

Five Star Quality Rating System for Medicare Advantage Plans

- For consumer education. Rates Medicare Advantage plans.[5]

Bridges to Excellence

- Incentive program for physicians focusing on quality measures, including incentive pay. Data submitted voluntarily.
- Patients can access website to find recognized clinicians.[6]

Leapfrog

- Hospital quality, safety and value rankings. For "those who use and pay for healthcare"; offers incentives and rewards.[7]

HCAHPS (Hospital Consumer Assessment of Healthcare Providers and Systems)

- The first nationwide standardized inpatient survey.[8]

J.D. Power and Associates

- Distinguished Hospital Program recognizes hospitals for service excellence[9]

NCQA (National Committee for Quality Assurance)

- Awards Multicultural Healthcare Distinction Seal to health plans and health organizations[10]

CAHPS (Consumer Assessment of Healthcare Providers and Systems)

- Comprehensive and standardized surveys for patients to evaluate their healthcare experiences. Program run by the US Agency for Healthcare Research and Quality (AHRQ)[11]

We physicians share in the desire to deliver better outcomes for our patients, so the pressure from society to achieve outcomes should be welcomed by us. Done well, the increased availability of data and measures should help us know whether we are delivering high-quality care and whether we are making improvements. We have an unprecedented capability to hold the mirror up to ourselves, and to discover and improve areas where we are not delivering as well as we could. A wealth of data is at our fingertips, so why not gather it, study it, and improve what we do? In the abstract, this sounds great, but what does it really mean for doctors? Will we have to work under a tyranny of arbitrary measurements? Or will the drive to measure outcomes actually help us be better physicians?

As you can probably tell, I am a strong advocate of the benefits of metrics. Used appropriately, they enhance communication and help clarify an organization's vision and goals. They motivate and build momentum. Metrics allow organizations to benchmark against the competition. Organizations in every field learn that they should measure what is important to them. In healthcare, putting the spotlight on quality and service goals, patient outcomes, and desired behaviors leads to better performance across the organization.

Without measurement and feedback, physicians think we are doing a great job. We sit in our offices and conscientiously conduct our individual practices based on what we have learned, believing we are delivering the best care possible. We accept that things can go wrong, and in many cases we can identify reasons beyond our control. In our busy practices, we often don't have much time to think about whether there is a different way to achieve better outcomes.

At SCPMG we found out by holding up the measurement mirror that there were many areas where we weren't as good as we thought—that others were doing things differently and achieving better outcomes. When I first assumed my role as executive medical director, our doctors boasted about how good we were. But when I asked in 2004, "What do we lead the country in?" no one could answer. We're now using measurements to get an accurate picture of our performance. Only then can the many physicians in our partnership hold each other accountable for delivering the caliber of healthcare that we believe in, and achieve the goals we have set out for ourselves.

Transparency and Value

Electronic medical records are a watershed event in contemporary medicine, and I discussed in the last chapter why they're so critical to delivering the best care and why they're inevitable at this point. As they become common in exam rooms and on hospital units, they usher in unprecedented transparency and accountability. Every aspect of a patient's condition, as well as every individual action taken by a healthcare provider, is recorded, viewable, and trackable. Mistakes or omissions are not as easily "lost" in an EMR as they could be in a paper chart.

It is possible to track decisions and outcomes on all levels: for whole systems, in regions, for particular patient groups, by hospitals, medical offices, primary care and specialty groups, and on down to individual physicians.[12] Ultimately much of the data that are collected will be shared externally with various agencies and made available to the general public. At SCPMG, we have had to come to terms with knowing that our actions, whether ultimately beneficial or not, are now exposed to greater scrutiny. We know that we will be held accountable in ways that were not possible in the past.

This kind of exposure can be unnerving. Yet transparency is regularly cited as a critical component of healthcare reform.[13] It is essential to improving the value we get from our healthcare dollars, and to the accountability of the healthcare delivery system and of the medical profession. There are ethical, economic, and quality reasons to create transparency and increase accountability.[14] We can no longer hide behind the veil of professional autonomy.

Public transparency of performance data was cited in the 2001 Institute of Medicine's report as necessary to the redesign of the healthcare system to deliver greater value. The report noted that patients should be able to make informed decisions when choosing doctors, hospitals and insurance plans.[15] Customers and purchasers demand it. Outcome transparency will drive increased value in the entire system.[16] Both price and outcome transparency will aid patients and purchasers by allowing them to make rational decisions about how best to use their healthcare dollars. Price transparency will also help us physicians to do the right thing for our patients. Currently, physicians often don't actually know what a given medication, procedure, or test costs our patients, in part because they could be signed up with one of any number of particular insurance plans with different coverage.

In fact, not only physicians, but also insurance companies, patients, the government and healthcare organizations themselves often don't know total costs or the component elements. Price is not a good indicator of value. It is common in US healthcare for physicians in the same organizational unit performing the same procedure to use very different and variably expensive devices, drugs, tests, and equipment, sometimes despite evidence that more expensive technology offers no advantages over less expensive technology. Physicians are often unaware of cost differences in technology purchased by hospital systems. A recent study has shown that there is a difference of $7,700 for back surgery and $6,900 for hip replacement between hospitals in the highest priced group and those in the lowest price group, even after adjusting for severity of illness, patient mix, and local payment rates for physicians.[17] Differences are just as stark internationally. Kaplan and Porter cite a comparison of the cost of the total joint replacement cycle. Although the margin to providers is similar, the average reimbursement in Germany and Sweden is approximately $8,500 compared to an average of $30,000 in the US.[18] There is little understanding of the sources of this variation, or of how, if at all, this variation relates to outcomes.

Wide variation in costs and prices, and the opaqueness of the sources of costs, have led organizations such as the University of Texas's MD Anderson Cancer Center to start to combine outcome measurements with a time-driven, activity-based costing system that takes into account all input resources and provides more accurate patient-level costs by medical condition.[19] This approach is viewed as necessary to prepare to move from fee-for-service to bundled reimbursement. It also gives the Center the ability to more accurately discern where the costs are coming from, and to identify ways to make a significant difference in overall costs while at the same time relating the various elements of care to outcomes. The pressures in our country for healthcare systems to provide greater value are definitely leading to more measurement, greater transparency, and by implication, greater accountability.

Using Physician Metrics to Move the Needle on Quality and Value

At SCPMG, we now have systematic and common measurement and the regular sharing of comparative data to focus us all on improving care. We have seen continuous improvement in measures throughout the system. Each medical center receives a monthly Vital Signs report detailing fifty measures of our goals. Believe it or not, this is a much more focused report than our earlier measurement approaches, when each facility had many individual metrics and unrelated data points. The system could not easily learn from these data as the measures were not comparable, and it was difficult to pick out the high performers in order to copy their successes and achieve better performance. Just as important, our physicians didn't see the data as meaningful or actionable and it didn't help drive quality improvements.

The Vital Signs report details how each of our medical centers performs on specific metrics, such as cancer screening goals for breast, colon and cervical cancer, lipid control for cardiovascular patients, hypertension control, and HbA1c control in diabetics. In addition to the all-important quality of care measures, we also measure service, access, affordability, and drug utilization patterns. Customer service metrics include the percentage of patients satisfied with their telephone access, physician communication, and whether patients have the opportunity to establish a bond with a primary caregiver.

SCPMG Strategic Goals	Data Period for Reported Rankings	Medical Center Ranking				
		MC1	MC2	MC3	MC4	MC5
Z-Score Composite	Y11 M03	2	11	1	9	5
Medicare 5-Star HEDIS	Y11 M03	3	3	3	3	1
Breast Cancer Screening	Y11 M02	4	12	6	13	3
Cervical Cancer Screening	Y11 M02	3	9	5	12	2
Colorectal Cancer Screening	Y11 M02	11	4	6	13	2
Glycohemoglobin Control in Diabetics	Y11 M02	10	12	8	11	7
Lipid Control (Diabetics)	Y11 M02	8	10	1	11	4

Table 1: *Sample of Vital Signs Executive Summary*

An executive summary of the Vital Signs report ranks our medical centers' performance. Doctors see this as a challenge, because they're competitive. Doctors were the students who always wanted to get A's and were willing to work for them. A doctor wants to learn, know, and achieve. The feedback about actual performance—on dimensions that are meaningful to physicians—taps in on that desire. Through the distribution of these reports, we hope to achieve focus, learning, innovation, and to impact behavior.

We also distribute a Clinical Strategic Goals (CSG) report monthly to each medical center, measuring performance in relation to targets and external benchmarks. (Most of the CSG data is also included in the Vital Signs report.) First and foremost, strategic goals are those that will save the most lives. They also include areas where we have the largest gaps from the HEDIS ninetieth percentile; and areas like well-baby care that aren't necessarily life-saving, but are hallmarks of quality healthcare. At present we have sixteen CSG "Imperatives," including measures like smoking cessation, timeliness of prenatal care, and cervical cancer screening for women ages twenty-one to sixty-four.

It is possible to drill right down to individual doctors' measures of their individual patient panel. We produce a Physician Quality Composite, which includes seven to eight metrics taken from HEDIS data, measured at the level of individual physicians. Doctors can see their own data and how they compare to the overall medical group. This is a powerful tool to enhance physicians' learning and improve quality of care.

Physician Ownership. I believe that physicians need to be active in developing and owning the metrics that make sense for the delivery of high-quality and high-value medicine. KP's approach to drug utilization measures is an example of how we achieve physician ownership. Our Drug Utilization Action Team (DUAT) is physician-led and includes members who are Kaiser Permanente pharmacists. Its purpose is to help our physicians understand and adopt appropriate prescribing practices. It works in concert with another physician-led team that explores best practice as decided by the evidence,[20] and determines which pharmaceuticals will be on our formulary.

DUAT releases a set of utilization metrics on a regular basis. Dr. Joel Hyatt, assistant medical director of SCPMG and the leader of DUAT, stresses that this approach is successful because it is led by physicians, and because the approach to prescribing is guided first by quality of care considerations, and only secondarily by cost (see box about how DUAT works), and because doctors have the final decision about which drug to prescribe for any individual patient. We develop measures that physicians feel are actionable, and provide the evidence so that individual doctors see their importance and the logic behind them, and can adjust their behavior to accomplish the ultimate purposes of high-quality and high-value medicine. For example, DUAT took measures to raise physicians' awareness of the nationwide problem that the prescription pain medication OxyContin is finding its way to the streets in increasing amounts, a very large concern in our Southern California communities.[21] In fact, fatal overdoses of prescription narcotics now claim more lives than traffic accidents.[22] DUAT drew our physicians' attention to OxyContin prescribing patterns. Figures 2 and 3 show the impact that such awareness had on subsequent prescribing patterns. We feel this is a win for our members and the communities we live in.

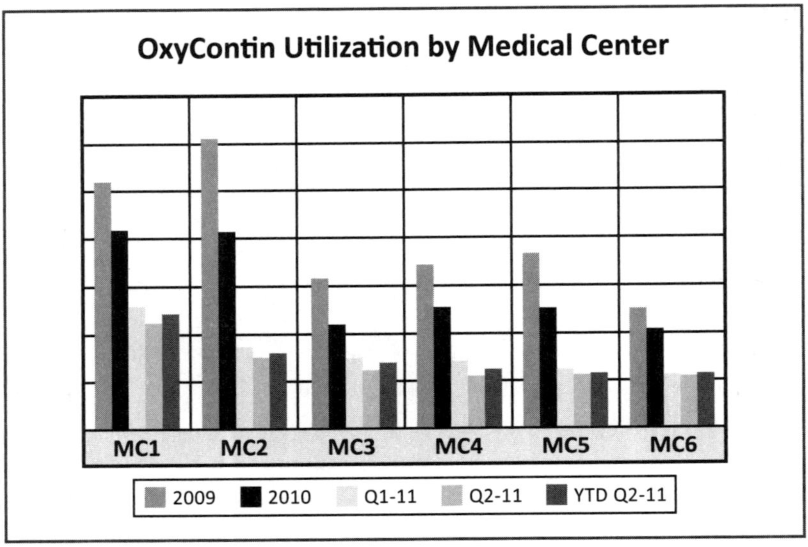

Figure 2: DUAT Data: OxyContin Utilization by Medical Center.
Table shows trends and does not show specific numbers for proprietary reasons.

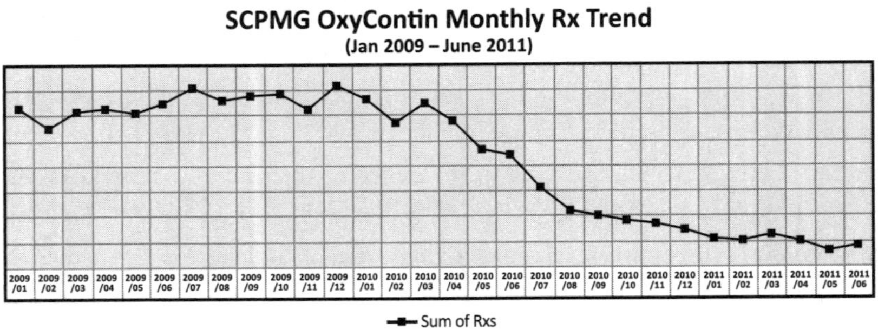

Figure 3: DUAT Data: SCPMG OxyContin Monthly Rx Trend.
Table shows trends and does not show specific numbers for proprietary reasons.

SCPMG's Drug Utilization Action Team

DUAT's purpose is to help our physicians understand and adopt appropriate prescribing practices. It is physician led: comprised of primary care and specialty care leaders, the head of the regional Pharmacy & Therapeutics (P& T) committee, pharmacy leaders, a medical group administrator, a health plan executive, as well as the regional chiefs of pediatrics, internal and family medicine.

Recommendations and Metrics:

- **Are Based on Evidence:** The primary criterion is efficacy and the secondary criterion is value. The first-line (preferred) drug is one that evidence shows is the most efficacious, and in some, but not all, cases is less costly than other drugs that have the same general level of efficacy. Second- and third-line drugs are identified and recommended if the preferred drugs don't work.

- **Maintain Physician Choice:** It is the physician's decision what drug to use for a particular patient.

- **Are Actionable:** DUAT metrics are not traditional high-level utilization metrics, but rather, are designed to be actionable and to address issues that physicians feel are important. Examples of DUAT measures:
    - the use of skeletal muscle relaxants for elderly patients, generally agreed to be a safety issue.
    - milligrams of OxyContin prescribed per person at a given facility, reflecting national concern that it too often finds its way onto the streets.
    - antibiotic usage with Moxifloxacin/Avelox for viral infections such as upper respiratory infection/viral bronchitis, an issue of concern because of severe side-effects and resistance.

- **Encourage Use of Preferred Drugs:** Metrics include the frequency of prescribing first-line drugs versus the others. Targets are not set for particular drugs. Physician judgment about what is best for a particular patient is paramount. Examining variation in these metrics that are distributed within our organization is a powerful way to get the discussion going, to further educate physicians, and to help shape behavior changes to adhere to evidence and to deliver value.

Using the Metrics. Dr. Jim DeFontes, head of Regional Perioperative Services, and physician director of Surgical Services in Orange County, describes some of the ways in which monthly surgical metrics are used to impact behavior and performance in a medical center. Under DeFontes's leadership, increasing emphasis has been focused on patient safety, which includes patient "never" events, surgical site infection rates, a Surgical Care Improvement Project (SCIP) composite score, and OR throughput. He goes over the measures with his perioperative team in Orange County each month, and with the operating room committee and the nursing teams in the ORs. They talk about performance and what can be done to improve the operating room workflow. The regional chiefs of service talk about the data with surgeons in their monthly meetings. DeFontes also meets regularly with senior leaders throughout the Southern California region. Tracking these metrics has contributed to a 30 percent increase in surgical output in the region since 2004. Our surgical backlog has been more than halved.

Choice of Metrics. HealthConnect lets us measure just about everything. But the software doesn't tell us what measures are important or what our targets should be. We have extremely intelligent people who are knowledgeable about the evidence, and who think about what to measure, how to slice the data, what to focus on, and how to present the data to motivate our doctors to accomplish the outcomes the partnership has decided are important. We don't set targets for everything, because some behaviors are more important than others. For example, DUAT has shifted its focus over time as its goals are met and new ones come to light. We know that goals that don't have anything to do with what doctors are really facing everyday may alienate them and won't help us deliver better healthcare. And even though physicians are determining the metrics, their rationale must be communicated persuasively to all of our doctors. Once we start looking at performance and translating it into the number of lives saved and the quality of work we do, people become very engaged.

Impact on Physicians. At SCPMG, the heightened transparency we all experienced has led to improved morale and improved performance. Both internal and external metrics say that our region is improving and leading the nation in many measures. Our national rankings have been a great source of pride to our entire system. We are in the top ten by HEDIS in areas such as cervical cancer screenings, cholesterol management, and comprehensive diabetes care, and are ranked number one in the US in controlling blood pressure in the elderly. "I now see the region living the KP promise and earnestly changing lives. The true focus on providing quality care by driving accountability has made tremendous changes. I now find myself singing our praises in the social events where I used to not discuss where I worked," notes Russell Lo Bue, RN, CEN, MBA, clinical director of Emergency Services, Downey Medical Center.

I know that many doctors will see this reliance on metrics and transparency as yet another assault on their autonomy, judgment, and clinical skills. Historically, physicians have mostly been reluctant and resistant to measurements and the transparency of data. After all, we are doctors—that means we know what's best for our patients. We've been tested, graded, and assessed in medical schools, internships, residencies, and fellowships, and now we physicians are going to be graded yet again? I'm not unsympathetic to the view that this is one more thing piled on our plates to add to the stress and pressure we deal with every day. I understand that some of us are insulted by a measurement approach, or see it as a lack of trust in our capabilities. But I don't agree.

Yes, we doctors are getting graded again. In all of the measures I've described, there are real numbers that track what each doctor, each clinic, each medical center has done. You can argue, "We never did this in the old days," and it's true. In the past, most doctors had no idea how well they were doing, except anecdotally or by reputation. Doctors couldn't get feedback about their actual performance the way we can now with data analysis. I am convinced by our experiences at SCPMG that seeing this kind of data and tracking how and what we are doing as compared to our colleagues helps us become more effective physicians. And that's the purpose.

In the past, most doctors had no idea how well they were doing, except anecdotally or by reputation. Doctors couldn't get feedback about their actual performance the way we can now with data analysis. I am convinced by our experiences at SCPMG that seeing this kind of data and tracking how and what we are doing as compared to our colleagues helps us become more effective physicians. And that's the purpose.

Dr. Ben Chu, the president of the Southern California Region, Kaiser Foundation Health Plan, Inc. & Hospitals, an internist and now the chair-elect designate of the American Hospital Association (AHA), chuckles understandingly when he says that we physicians almost go through the five stages of death and dying as we learn to deal with metrics and having this level of transparency in our work. Eventually, doctors find acceptance and a resolve to figure out how to work with it.

Instead of focusing on what is being done to us, we doctors should think about how we can take charge of the reason we went into medicine–to make a difference in people's lives.

We know that it's still overwhelming for physicians. That's one of the reasons why we have assembled a team around the doctor, so that they can share and meaningfully contribute to the workload. It's also one of the reasons why doctors have to get more involved and be part of designing a better system for everyone. Instead of focusing on what is being done to us, we doctors should think about how we can take charge of the reason we went into medicine —to make a difference in people's lives.

Metrics as the Basis for System Improvement

My discovering, at my first national meeting as SCPMG's medical director, that the Southern California region's breast cancer screening rates metric was the lowest in the Kaiser Permanente system became the germ of our intense work on making sure that we became leaders in prevention and treatment quality in many areas. This required changing not only the behavior of our physicians, but of the entire system in which we operated.

We realized that we needed to improve quickly. We set a goal of 80 percent for breast cancer screening in the first year, found champions to lead the improvement, did an in-depth analysis of our screening program and started to work on details such as throughput/mammograms per hour, hours of operation, number of mammogram machines and technicians needed, outreach, missed opportunity reports, and panel management. We put in a quality performance incentive for our breast screening clinical strategic goal for both our doctors and ancillary staff workers.

We all knew that this was important. Breast cancer is a very important issue for women and their families, and a very emotional one. It is essential to diagnose this disease early so it can be cured. Early detection improves quality/health outcomes, decreases the need for advanced and often toxic treatment, and decreases cost. In short, it is a high-value strategy. Two years ago we moved to the top of the nation in breast cancer screening in women over age fifty-two.

Our breast cancer screening focus came at a time when we were starting to understand that it wasn't enough for our physicians to provide good care.

Rather, we needed to provide great care, especially in the area of prevention. We would have to improve the processes throughout our whole system. The healthcare status of our members depends on continually improving our ability to perform as an integrated system. To guide the changes in how we operate, we rely heavily on measurements, which we use to detect opportunities for improvement, learn the impact of the changes we make, and to continually improve outcomes.

As one example of our approach, KPSC developed and put in place a comprehensive measurement-based Hospital Acquired Infection (HAI) and Hospital Acquired Condition (HAC) prevention program, which has several focuses, including Central Line Associated Blood Stream Infections (CLABSI), Ventilator Acquired Pneumonia (VAP), Surgical Site Infections (SSI), Retained Foreign Objects (RFO) and Hospital Acquired Pressure Ulcers (HAPU). Hospital safety is a nation-wide problem. The Institute for Healthcare Improvement (under former president and CEO Don Berwick's tenure) initiated the 100,000 Lives Campaign in 2004 (and later the 5 Million Lives Campaign) as a result of the Institute of Medicine report, *To Err is Human*, which estimated that ninety-eight thousand people died every year in American hospitals because of medical injuries.[23]

Hospital safety is an area where we in SCPMG and our co-workers in the Kaiser Foundation Hospitals organization have aligned around a common strategy and sense of urgency. Doctors work in concert with nurses and other members of Unit-Based Teams in each hospital to improve safety. Both physicians and non-physicians in each hospital champion local efforts, share best practices, and are accountable for progress to the goal. Such efforts are only possible when there are good measures in place. John August, Executive Director, Coalition of Kaiser Permanente Unions, and our partner in the Coalition of Kaiser Permanente Unions + Kaiser Permanente collaboration, talks about the importance of all stakeholders developing an understanding of the science of performance improvement, a science based on continuous measurement of outcomes, and introduction and testing of process changes designed to improve them.

For the reduction of CLABSI, for example, we first implemented best practices from the Centers for Disease Control and Prevention (CDC) and the Institute for Healthcare Improvement (IHI), as well as additional findings from the evidence-based literature. Then our teams used the common "Plan-Do-Study-Act" (PDSA) process improvement methodology to further improve our processes and drive down the HAI and HAC rates. Now, such practices as the establishment of consistent dressing change practices and time intervals, as well as two-person dressing changes, has led to our regional rate of CLABSIs in the intensive care unit to fall 20 percent in one year. Our 2010 performance was .69/1000 line days compared to the NHSN average of 1.48/1000 line days. Our careful measurement of improvement in outcomes provides confirmation of the value of the approaches we have put into place, as well as targets for improvement.

Similarly, the problem of VAP was approached by first taking the recommendations from the American Thoracic Society, CDC Guidelines, IHI and other recommendations in the clinical literature. These were further enhanced with more literature reviews and our performance improvement process findings. We have reduced the VAP rate of occurrence by 33 percent from 2009 to 2010, with six of our hospitals having zero VAPs in the last twenty-four months.

Metrics align the purposes of the various healthcare providers and keep us all focused on the radar screen so that everything we do points to high-quality healthcare. They guide the improvement of our processes to reduce the frustration that comes from lack of coordination and wasted time, energy and resources. They allow healthy internal and external competition. They allow the development of learning forums where exchange of information can occur, and where people can learn how others are able to achieve better outcomes, and where the culture of "not invented here" goes away.

High-quality performance and value for the healthcare dollar are the gold at the end of the rainbow. Metrics make it easy to say what has been accomplished. This leads to an entire organization being more satisfied and proud. At KPSC we use "Did You Know" cards to share our accomplishments internally and externally. Through measurable accomplishments and metrics that are shared throughout the state and the nation, external branding has improved and everyone feels proud to be part of the system. For example, based on Kaiser Permanente's successful breast cancer screening program, a newspaper ad was developed saluting KP women in Southern California for being diligent about their breast cancer screenings. The ad also encouraged all women to be proactive in getting mammograms. We're proud that we have metrics and accomplishments that show we're doing everything we can to make it more likely that the people under our care will live long and happy lives.

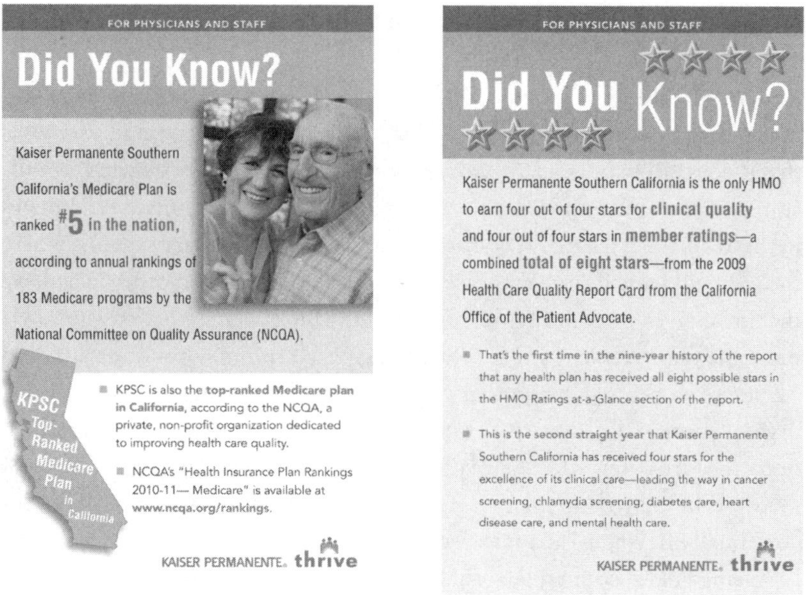

Figure 4: *Did You Know? Cards*

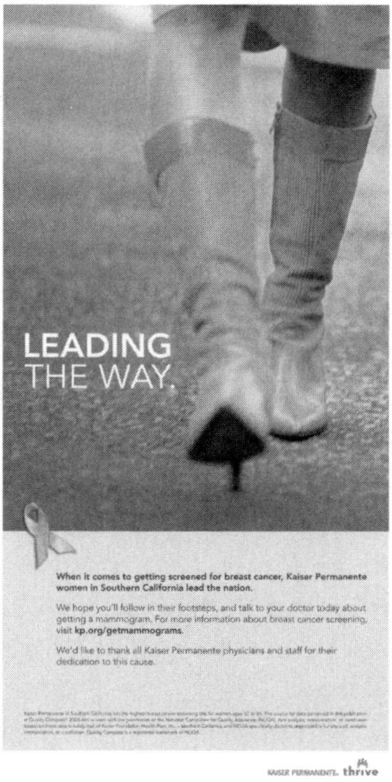

Figure 5: *Leading the Way Newspaper ad*

Quality Performance Incentives and Accountability

You may be reading this and wondering whether any of this pertains to you if you do not work in an integrated healthcare system. My simple answer is that it does. Reimbursement and reporting requirements are demanding outcomes metrics and improvement, and aligning quality performance incentives in this direction. There is pressure to build accountable care systems where the various elements of healthcare delivery are integrated in order to achieve the advantages of coordination and process improvement as measured by outcome improvement and increased value. More and more of us will find ourselves working in integrated systems, even if these are not all under one organizational roof. Doctors' work and income streams, and their patients' outcomes are being affected by these trends. We can either become actively involved in improving the systems we work with or we will find ourselves continually having to adapt to requirements not of our own making.

Being held accountable to the outcomes of a complicated system of care delivery, much of which is beyond our individual control, may seem both unfair and distasteful to physicians. We trained to deliver high-quality care, and doing that in today's world leaves us with little time and energy to worry about making improvements, figuring out how to deliver greater value, and achieving what may seem to us to be arbitrary outcomes. The changes that are being made may seem to us to make it harder, not easier, to provide good care. What's in this for us?

You may be thinking: fifty metrics in the Vital Signs report and sixteen Critical Strategic Goals? Doesn't this just totally deflect the attention of the system away from what's important? Indeed, many in SCPMG have asked me why there are so many metrics and so many initiatives. They ask which of these do you want us to concentrate on? My answer is that we need to attend to all of them—not the right wing or level wheel, but the entire plane and person. These metrics are not optional. They are the measures of what we do every day. They measure the outcomes of our care. Each physician individually doesn't need to shoulder the burden of figuring out how we can deliver better care. But at SCPMG, I do expect that we will all act on what has been learned about approaches that will improve our outcomes.

So get real, Jeff, my colleagues might say. What's the incentive for us to change our behavior when we feel we're already doing great work? Aren't we talking about a long, slow process of introducing change and overcoming resistance? And besides, when you introduce "value" into the equation, are you asking us to deliver lower quality care? These questions are why we have to carefully examine the incentives in our healthcare systems to ensure that they are aligned with quality outcomes. The highest quality patient care is what all of us—physicians, hospitals, payers, and especially patients—are trying to achieve.

Physicians, like other professionals, are incentivized by many factors. Having the conditions and support in place to deliver high-quality care without constraints and interference motivates many of us. Other motivators include achieving respect from colleagues, learning and improving, and helping patients be healthier. Indeed, all of these motivating factors have guided our many physician leaders throughout SCPMG during the past eight years, as we have led change designed to deliver high-value healthcare in today's challenging environment.

Although being a physician may be a labor of love and give us professional pride, it also provides our livelihoods. We want to ensure that we are fairly paid, and indeed we shape our professional activities to achieve financial, as well as professional, satisfaction. It is for this reason that I believe that financial incentives for quality outcomes have a role in healthcare.

Many take the opposite view. They worry that incentives can be perverse and can lead to bad trade-offs that sacrifice care and quality in order to reduce costs or increase revenue to achieve personal or organizational gain. Some may even see incentives as not belonging in a professional setting, believing that any administrative or economic concerns degrade and distort the value and autonomy of a professional.

My perspective is that throughout the US, the value delivered by our healthcare systems and by the physicians who are a part of them is hampered because financial incentives are misaligned with outcomes. This is starting to change. For example, the quality ratings received by Medicare Advantage health insurance plans from such measures as HEDIS, CAHPS and others are now tied to bonus payments, as mandated by the healthcare reform legislation. Plans that receive a five-star rating receive bonus payments up to 5 percent that can be ploughed into increased benefits or returned as reduced premiums. KPSC and several other Kaiser Permanente regions were among the nine systems to get the full five-star rating in 2011.[24] I believe these ratings are because of the emphasis we have placed on quality measures and outcomes.

At SCPMG, we have found that small incentives for quality outcomes, used carefully, can help to reinforce changes aimed at delivering better care to our members, and can heighten focus on achieving goals. We attach these incentives to our medical group's important quality outcomes and strategically important initiatives to enhance their salience.

Some of our physicians have reacted quite negatively to the idea of quality-based incentives, seeing them as a threat. They instead focus on the chance of not getting the incentive as a take-away rather than on the opportunity to get rewarded for high performance. Quality incentives motivate, but they also frighten people because they require performance and accountability.

The majority of our physicians have responded quite well to the notion that we are incentivizing the things that align with our vision. All of our physicians participate in a pay-for-quality-performance system. The quality performance incentives are additional to base compensation and are aligned with specific department, medical center, and regional goals. We do not put our physicians in competition with each other for dollars. The dollars involved are not a large amount; in fact, they are so small that some don't even notice the incremental pay. But physicians do not want to "fail"—especially in something as critical as the quality of care—so many work hard to get them.

We're learning a lot about how quality outcome incentives fit in with the building of a high-performance system. A few of the things we have learned:

1) *Provide incentives in areas that improve quality and achieve operational efficiencies.* Incentives should be focused on ways to increase value. Our quality incentives to increase colorectal screening are an example. This area was generally accepted as a high priority. Nationwide, colorectal cancer is an area that consumes an inordinate amount of resources—with each advanced stage cancer costing up to $1.3 million in treatment. Patient outcomes are quite poor due to the poor prognosis for late stage disease. Our efforts to increase early detection have included enabling our members to return stool samples by mail for fecal immunochemical testing (FIT). We have also increased access to colonoscopies. Based on the evidence, the department of anesthesiology is now delivering propofol anesthesia rather than Versed. This has led to easier and quicker recovery for patients and allowed for quicker turnover in the endoscopy GI suites. Most importantly, it has greatly increased our colonoscopy screening rates. The evidence continues to show that colonoscopy saves lives.[25] Our focus on early detection and the resulting rapid treatment has translated to a decrease in the number of stage four cancers from 18 percent to 12 percent, and improved survival.

2) *Incentives have to be based on good metrics that physicians believe are valid and important indicators of high-quality care.* The NCQA Diabetes Recognition Program for physicians includes eleven measures.[26] If doctors have more than twenty-five diabetics in their panels, they are eligible to apply for this distinction, which recognizes the highest standards of diabetes care. We electronically gather and submit data to NCQA for any of our physicians who want to take part. Although we do incent our doctors to participate, this award is seen as a real indicator of the highest quality diabetes care. Additionally, this award gives physicians some credits toward board recertification.

3) *Physicians need to believe that the system can be improved so that the quality incentive is achievable.* Our incentives have generally been in the context of systematic organizational quality improvement efforts—efforts to create the processes to achieve the very metrics that are being incentivized. For example, we have incentivized the improvement of surgical throughput in a number of different frequent surgeries, including cataracts, hernia, total joint replacement, and bariatric surgery—surgical domains where we had experienced backlogs and considerable expense. We know that surgical productivity depends on many factors and many different team members coming together with efficient processes.

Many different process improvement efforts have focused on simultaneously achieving the metrics of surgery quality and safety (e.g., no wrong-site surgeries, antibiotics administered pre-operatively, no retained foreign objects, etc.), and on throughput metrics such as timely room turnover and on-time pre-surgery team coordination. Physicians were heavily involved in making the changes. Once the metrics were put in place and the processes were designed to make it possible to achieve the targets, physicians became quite comfortable with goals to improve throughput. The quality incentive program had worked.

In short, incentives should be in areas that are closely connected to the vision to deliver high-quality, high-value healthcare. At SCPMG, all of our specialty areas have been asked to identify high-impact areas of change that will lead to our being best in class in quality and value. Our physicians have been actively involved in creating the vision, in determining the areas of focus and the metrics for success, and in defining the changes required to get to our desired outcomes. Quality incentives are one approach to motivating such change. Based on the right metrics and accompanied by efforts to improve the system, they provide focus and help shine the light on outstanding performance.

Trend	Implications for Physicians	Am I effectively dealing with this trend now?
Healthcare and Its Outcomes are Being Measured		
	1. Accountability of doctors and all healthcare workers to internal and external stakeholders 2. Pay based on measurable outcomes, not volume of activity 3. Scrutiny, transparency, and exposure of individual physicians' performance 4. Reimbursement and reporting requirements demand outcomes metrics and improvement	
Aggregated Data Have Many Uses		
	1. Aggregated patient data used to improve practice and increase physician awareness 2. Metrics play a large role in system and process improvement. 3. Metrics enable incentive pay structures, which can build high-quality performance.	

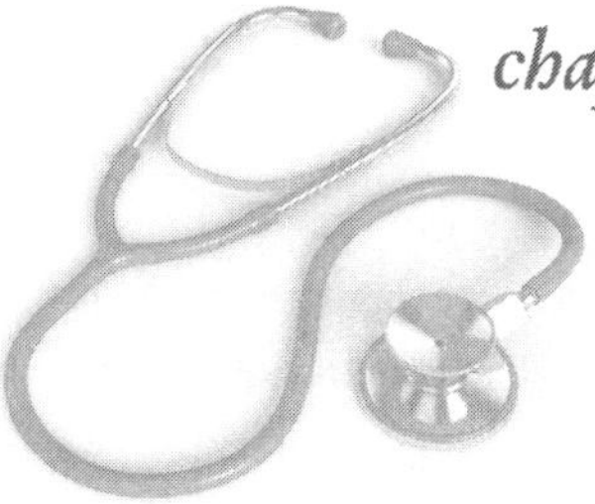

chapter six

Keeping Up to Date: Evidence-Based Practice and Continuing Medical Education

As new doctors, after completing many years of training and study and passing our boards, we enter practice with our knowledge at a peak. Without diligence, it can quickly go downhill from there. At the same time that we are accumulating experience and clinical expertise by providing patient care, we are challenged to keep up with rapid developments in the scientific basis of our practices and in the treatments that become available. For example, genetic testing and molecular diagnostic testing in areas such as breast and colon cancer and cystic fibrosis continue to increase in scope and importance. Pharmacogenetics and the rapidly developing field of personalized medicine have profound and powerful possibilities for our patients. We see examples such as Herceptin having significant response rates against breast tumors only for those positive for the Her2neu receptor. New technologies and techniques such as robotics employed for minimally invasive surgery, and endoscopic and laparoscopic surgeries such as natural orifice transluminal endoscopic surgery, continue to develop. Biomedical knowledge advances have led to many new treatment possibilities, and there is continuous infusion of new drugs and enhanced imaging technologies, each bringing their own contingencies and initial uncertainties about efficacy, safety, and cost benefit.

New knowledge often comes in the form of new methodologies and technologies, accompanied by claims being made by their proponents, inventors, and detractors. The most effective of these will be translated into new ways of practicing medicine. Randomized blind trials and comparative effectiveness research provide knowledge about the efficacy of various treatments and ways of delivering care. As individual practitioners, we have to find our path through the barrage of new claims and possibilities. We have to make sense of all this new knowledge and, where appropriate, incorporate it into our work.

Knowledge advances challenge the ways we were taught to practice medicine, but research indicates that we physicians change our practice patterns slowly and with healthy skepticism. There is often a large gap between our practices and what science has shown as evidence-based practice guidelines. On the one hand, adults in the US receive only about 50 percent of the recommended processes for care, whether preventive, acute, or chronic.[1] On the other hand, there is overuse of many treatments in situations where they are not indicated. For example, even though the American Heart Association and the American College of Cardiology revised the guidelines on angioplasty and stenting after a 2006 US National Heart, Lung, and Blood Institute study (the Occluded Artery Trial), a recent study detailed in the *Archives of Internal Medicine* shows continued overuse of angioplasty and stents for stable coronary patients showing no evidence of heart attack.[2]

In many areas the knowledge base needed to guide practice has been scant. Many guidelines and approaches are based on "expert opinion." However, the pace of knowledge growth has accelerated, and the evidence base for medical practice is growing rapidly. If you're just now finishing medical school, you should assume that the way you practice medicine in the future is likely to be vastly different than how you were taught.

Physicians are expected to be up-to-date in our knowledge and to evolve our practices according to the evidence. The trend is to evaluate us and pay us for adherence to best practice, and for the clinical outcomes of our patients, not just for volume of activity. New capabilities for measurement and reporting mean that our work will be transparent—to patients, colleagues, and other stakeholders. There will be less room for idiosyncratic individualism on the part of physicians, and more of our practices will be prescribed by evidence-based standards. To use society's healthcare dollars wisely, we must weigh the efficacy as well as the costs and benefits of various approaches, discard practices that are ineffective, and choose lower cost alternatives that are equally or more efficacious.

This raises many questions for us. How do we stay abreast of rapidly developing knowledge and still have time for our clinical practice? How do we team with each other to combine different knowledge specialties so that we're efficiently bringing the right combination of expertise to bear on the particular individual we are treating? How do we make sure that we incorporate new knowledge in a way that enables us to use sound clinical judgment to address the individual differences of our patients?

Doctors making treatment decisions may be acting on information several years out of date—not out of malice, but just out of habit or lack of time. Many of us may resist changing the way we practice, and claim the new evidence-based approaches don't fit our particular patients. We may be distrustful of new approaches that we feel are not sufficiently proven. Or we may not believe these changes are in our best interests financially or otherwise. Yet not responding to new evidence puts patients and doctors at risk.

Physicians and patients alike are becoming aware that in the US there is a wide disparity in treatment depending on where patients are treated and who treats them. Where in the nation you live shouldn't matter when it comes to your medical treatment, but it often does, resulting in inequities in quality and in resources consumed. The Dartmouth Atlas of Healthcare has been documenting the capricious nature of medical treatment in the US for several years and the impact this has on both quality of care and its cost. One report drawing upon the Atlas data noted that Medicare patients in the highest-spending regions spend more days in the hospital, have more frequent doctor visits, and get more MRIs and CT scans than similar patients in the lowest-spending regions. The data shows that regional factors account for 70 percent of the cost differential, far surpassing health factors, income, and race.[3]

A 2009 article by Dr. Atul Gawande in *The New Yorker* documented widely divergent spending on Medicare recipients in El Paso and McAllen, Texas, two cities in counties with very similar public health profiles. El Paso spends half as much as McAllen ($7,504 vs. $15,000 per person, respectively) with no difference in outcomes. In fact, McAllen's five largest hospitals performed worse than El Paso's on most of the twenty-five metrics of care that Medicare uses to rank hospitals.[4] Local practice patterns account for this difference. Attending to the evidence should help reduce these disparities. Even more important, it should help us make sure that we carry out our responsibility to ensure that the resources consumed in delivering healthcare go toward efficacious treatments and deliver high value to our patients and society.[5]

Evidence-based practice (EBP) is critical to continually improve the capabilities of healthcare. Continuing medical education (CME), done well, keeps doctors attuned to the latest and best research and thinking in our fields. Without evidence and continual education, we get stuck in a time warp, practicing what and how we were taught in school, even years after we've graduated. EBP is an approach that can enhance physicians' clinical expertise and experience by combining them with the best available research data and information. But it should not be a prescription for a cold, unthinking, unfeeling application of scientific knowledge. With EBP, doctors draw upon the latest and most scientifically validated research studies to inform their decision making with respect to particular patients and conditions.

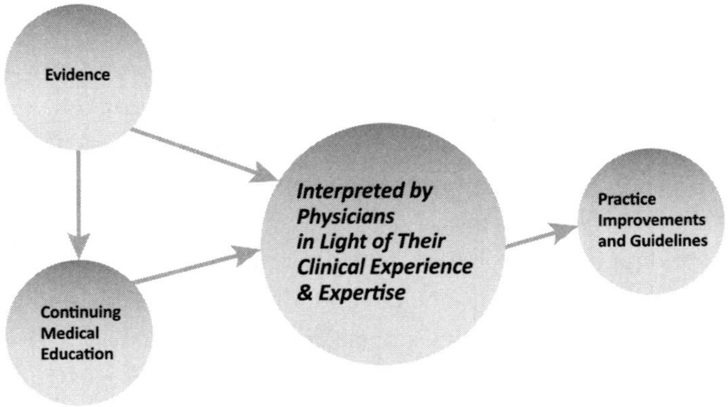

Figure 1: *Flow of Evidence Into Practice*

Making the Evidence Accessible

Keeping up with the evidence will take intentional strategies, and we'll have to work together. PubMed, the service of the National Center for Biotechnology Information, touts on its homepage (http://www.ncbi.nlm.nih.gov/pubmed) that it offers over 20 million individual biomedical citations. MEDLINE, which is one part of PubMed, indexes over fifty-five thousand journals worldwide in thirty-nine languages. There were approximately seven hundred thousand references added to MEDLINE in 2010 alone.[6] As practicing physicians, how can we possibly keep up with this torrent of information? We are leading hectic lives to begin with, dealing with the many predictable and unpredictable aspects of treating our patients, receiving an avalanche of journals, or wondering if a colleague giving us advice is aware of the latest developments for the given situation. Keeping up with knowledge takes time and energy we may not have.

The time-consuming nature of each of us independently scouring the original literature to consider the validity of new studies that might impact a patient should not be underestimated. Having access to secondary sources, including pre-assessed evidence-based summaries, practice guidelines, and protocols, is crucial for today's physicians. Fortunately there are some excellent consolidations of current knowledge, but even these are imposing. The Cochrane Library (http://www.thecochranelibrary.com), the *ACP Journal Club*, and *Evidence-Based Medicine* are three well-known resources for medical practitioners. The Cochrane Library is a collection of several databases, including the Cochrane Database of Systematic Reviews, which features over five thousand reviews and over two thousand protocols. The total number of published articles in all of its databases numbers over seven hundred forty thousand.[7] The *ACP Journal Club*, a monthly feature of the *Annals of Internal Medicine*, consolidates findings from over one hundred clinical journals on internal medicine. *Evidence-Based Medicine* appraises and summarizes findings from over one hundred journals and approximately fifty thousand articles yearly on internal and primary medicine.

To help physicians stay up to date, various national specialty associations, such as the American Academy of Neurology[8] or the American College of Radiology,[9] issue guidelines and best practices that build on the evidence. And, we're getting our information in new ways—not just online, but via smartphone apps too! The *ACP Journal Club* is available in an online version, which includes

Evidence-Based Practice: Two Physicians' Views

Dr. Brian Nguyen, Physician Director of Clinical Strategic Goals Optimization

"We're adopting things so much faster than we used to. Ten to twenty years ago if a new medication or algorithm for blood pressure came out, it took a much longer time for adoption. Now, when there are evidence-based practices published on how to better manage blood pressure, we adopt it very quickly. What used to take years now may only take months. The field of medicine changes exponentially. It's a struggle for physicians on the front line to get everything. There is so much to know. Each new class of physicians knows more or knows something more current. How can human beings keep the information in their heads and manage every nuance? You have to rely on technology to help remind you of all the things you need to attend to. On the other hand, there may be a peak of how many clinical pop-up reminders can be foisted on physicians, especially if they can't validate the information quickly at the time of seeing the patient. They may become jaded."

Dr. Todd Sachs, Chief of Surgery for West Los Angeles

"Physicians are trained to make evidence-based decisions. However, we need to see data before making changes. It's part of our DNA. Dr. Michael Kanter (SCPMG's regional medical director of Quality and Clinical Analysis) has pushed to ensure that the most recent evidence is readily available to all our physicians through many sources. For instance, we have educational time to make sure we continue to evaluate the evidence. Also, a variety of data is sent to us and we receive computerized alerts when there is a change in medication warnings. We work quickly through the day, so these alerts are very helpful and serve as a safety check. We are also fortunate to exchange ideas and knowledge among our surgeons, often centered around prospective reviews of our cases. It's fantastic."

the last ten years of articles from the journal. Hospital medical libraries are closing because information is available on the Internet twenty-four/seven. Smartphones give doctors the Internet and apps plus mobility. Apps for the iPhone and other smartphones aim to help with symptoms, diagnosis, drug interactions, and clinical information.

Being Part of a Knowledge Network

Even with best practice guidelines, knowledge summaries, and mobile apps, there is still a lot for individual physicians to keep up with as we try to manage a busy practice. In today's world, physicians need to be well connected to a knowledge support network that provides easy and quick access to the latest scientific findings and their implications for practice. Frankly, one of the benefits of working in a large medical system, whether SCPMG or another large group, is that it has the ability to distill a lot of the research for member physicians so they have more time to practice medicine. A large system makes it easier to share knowledge. And it makes it more possible to involve physicians in interpreting the evidence, discussing practice guidelines, and generating new evidence. One example showing the importance of the network is that hundreds of private practice physicians are teaming up with Providence Health and Services of Southern California, a large hospital system, to share and analyze data and find best practices.[10]

KPSC consists of thirteen medical centers with more than six thousand physicians practicing medicine over approximately twenty thousand square miles. That's a large number of highly expert physicians striving to stay up-to-date while providing high-quality and responsive care, and trying to have work-life balance. Each medical center has a chief of service for each medical, surgical, and subspecialty area, and one of the thirteen is the regional chief of service for the specialty. The chiefs for a given specialty meet regularly as a group to discuss and debate trends in the literature, to review evidence, and to identify current best practices. Often these SCPMG specialty groups share knowledge nation-wide, across the Permanente Medical Groups of the eight regions of Kaiser Permanente. The evidence is shared and debated among all the doctors in that specialty through yearly symposia, web-based presentations and at their monthly departmental meetings.

Interaction between physicians in interpreting new evidence is critical in determining its significance. Aware that one-time events and lectures don't generally change behavior, Dr. Marc Klau, the regional chief of our head and neck surgeons, started a monthly series of webinars for doctors in his specialty so that they could interact on a whole host of pressing topics and issues. The webinars are led by a physician expert, who is joined by one or two discussants on the call. Physicians viewing and listening can chat and ask questions. Attendance at the webinars is growing, and it's becoming the new norm. The recorded webinars are also now archived and available via an intranet site. Through such interactions, the specialty moves toward common, up-to-date, evidence-based practices and beliefs about effective care. While practice guidelines should never replace a physician's judgment or decree what needs to be done in any individual case, this ability to discuss clinical issues and learn together is essential to advancing our practice.

Our physicians also get involved with specific medical issues even before they are in the literature. When they get together with their specialty groups to discuss, argue, and study the available evidence, they often identify holes in the knowledge and suggest new research areas. Frequently they become involved in investigating these questions using our own KP data, which can then yield new literature about the disease or issue in question. They contribute patient data to registries, which allow us to do comparative effectiveness studies of drugs, devices, and therapy pathways. For example, we investigated the pros and cons of various joint prostheses from a quality and cost perspective, and our urologists have investigated the appropriate screening tests for microscopic hematuria and whether some patients can safely avoid cystoscopy and unnecessary radiation from CT scans. Many of us become involved in clinical trials, leading to greater understanding and acceptance of the knowledge that is yielded and its limitations, and preparing us to introduce new practice should it turn out to be more effective. Typically, the first question our physicians ask is, "What's the evidence?" Now, not only do they spend time together thinking it through, in many cases they also help create it.

Ownership of the practice guidelines is critical to acceptance and behavioral change by our highly trained and experienced physicians. Advancing our practice is only possible if the physicians themselves translate the evidence into practice guidelines. An example of this is a change that our urologists have made in the use of Lupron to treat prostate cancer. Our physicians were using this very expensive and aggressive hormonal therapy and had concerns about whether it was being used effectively. Our regional chief of Urology, Dr. Ron Loo, worked with our pharmacy analysis group to track its impact and look at contingencies by analyzing HealthConnect data. As a result of this investigation, urologists are now adjusting Lupron dosage based on levels of testosterone in the patient, resulting in greater efficacy and fewer negative side-effects. Not only did our urologists change their practice, they also contributed knowledge to the broader medical community.[11] This has led to great pride in the practice.

Given the demonstrated power of sharing and discussing among physicians, additional links are being forged to further information and research and to build community among practitioners across all of the Permanente Medical Groups. For example, all eight regional chiefs of gastroenterology nationwide come together regularly, meeting bi-monthly via conference calls and face-to-face twice a year. These efforts contribute to bringing together 285 gastroenterologists in KP nationwide into a community of practice, who individually and as a group review and catalyze research and translate it into practice. They share best practices, develop consensus guidelines, and improve operational effectiveness through this forum. For example, they have been able to dramatically increase colorectal cancer screening rates by focusing on two modalities of screening: FIT (fecal immunochemical testing) and colonoscopy. A pilot study done in Southern California found that using propofol, although a more expensive anesthetic agent to administer, can be cost effective by increasing colonoscopy throughput (with fewer medication side effects and enhanced recovery) while improving quality, outcomes, and patient satisfaction. Dr. Alexander Lee, the regional chief of Gastroenterology, has been a proponent of the propofol model and helped implement it not only in Southern California but in other regions as well, thus translating findings into practice.

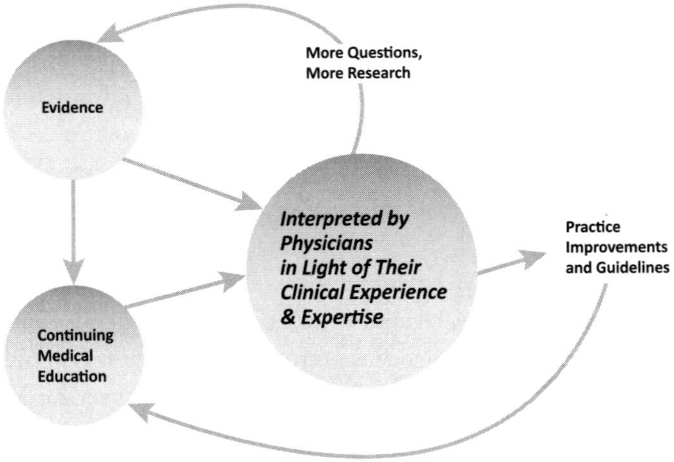

Figure 2: *Physician Leadership in Generating and Incorporating Evidence Into Practice*

Patients Come with Information

The US is one of the few nations that allows direct-to-consumer advertising of prescription pharmaceuticals. Americans are inundated with television and print ads, especially for new (and expensive) prescription drugs. That very often translates into requesting these in a doctor's office. "I want that little purple pill for my heartburn."

This is another reason why we doctors need up-to-date information to decide if the drug actually is the most appropriate one to treat our patient. Studying the results of clinical trials and understanding what we know and don't know about a drug is a demanding task. Here again, it is helpful to be part of a system or a network that analyzes data and can give us information. The information backs up our decisions to prescribe or not prescribe a drug and provides the basis for a discussion with the patient about which drug is best and why.

In a similar vein, where I live, Los Angeles, seems to be blanketed at present with billboards advertising lap band surgery. I've even seen lap band ads targeting teenagers in my local paper. As we all know, obesity is rampant. Many patients, convinced by the ads, come into our offices requesting lap band surgery. The problem is there have not been any studies on long-term lap band safety and efficacy. In comparison, there is a wealth of evidence about traditional gastric bypass surgery, including both short-term and long-term consequences. This is an instance where we physicians have to deal with the uncertainty of not knowing for sure whether a treatment that has been released will be safe and efficacious in the long term. I hope that this does not turn out to be a situation similar to bone marrow transplantation for breast cancer, which was approved too soon, and resulted in even more pain and suffering for women.

At SCPMG, it is our strong belief that the use of drugs is a clinical decision that should be made by physicians. To foster the most appropriate prescribing of pharmaceuticals by our large physician partnership, Dr. Joel Hyatt worked with our chiefs of service and with KP Pharmacy Operations to create the Drug Utilization Action Team (DUAT) to focus on and promote best practices through evidence-based drug use (this was described more fully in chapter five). The regional team is composed of physician leaders from primary care and all of our specialties, working with a pharmacy leader, a health plan leader and a hospital administrator. The pharmacy presents the evidence; decisions about what drugs to put on the formulary and what will be first line (recommended) and second and third line drug treatments for various conditions are made by the team. No drugs are prohibited—as we realize that there are many individual differences in our patients that may respond best to third-level drugs or even off-formulary drugs. But our commitment as a medical group is that we will prescribe appropriate drugs based on the evidence. We believe that this delivers the greatest quality of care and the greatest value.

Historically our profession has largely relied on pharmaceutical and device companies to educate us about new treatment technologies. We have relied on the very organizations that have the most to gain financially by quickly influencing us to adopt their products. Many of these products represent stunning advances in efficacy, ease of use, and quality of life. Yet others are minimal improvements over what has gone before, and most arrive with a high price tag and incomplete knowledge about their impact on different populations of patients and about their side effects. Physicians need support in looking critically at these advances to determine how and when they should be applied. Do they work for children? Do they work in combination with other treatments and drugs or is there an undesirable interaction? Are they more efficacious than other treatments that are less expensive? What about off-label prescribing? Provigil, the drug approved to treat narcolepsy and shift sleep disorders, has also been prescribed off-label for generalized fatigue and depression. At SCPMG, we saw from the data that we were using it too frequently, so we put in guidelines for use and added notifications in our online physician ordering entry system to alert doctors to the various issues as they are ordering the drug. It was our most prescribed non-formulary drug. And yet we knew very little about its safety or efficacy for off-label use.

Consider the case of Vioxx, a drug that has now been withdrawn. It cost ten times as much as similar drugs, and it was marketed everywhere. Our doctors started questioning its safety, took a hard look at it, and Kaiser Permanente physicians used it substantially less than others in the medical community. When we crunched numbers and information from our pharmacy database, SCPMG became one of the sources pointing to its association with heart attacks. I'm proud to say that our actions helped to take an unsafe drug off of the market. Just as important, I'm proud that we provide our physicians with a mechanism to raise concerns about drugs, that we carefully scrutinize claims about the efficacy and safety of new treatments, and that we regularly share the findings with our physicians who translate them into new practice guidelines. I believe this gives our physicians greater peace of mind—they're not alone in keeping track of the changing knowledge base underpinning healthcare today. It makes it easier to have the tough conversation with a demanding patient. And I believe it leads to higher quality and safer care for our patients. We are able to help the doctors in our system do what is right for the patient.

The importance of such a safety net for us and our patients is clear and the need is continual. For example, the anticonvulsant medication gabapentin was developed to treat epilepsy, but is now also prescribed for migraine headaches, hot flashes, smoking cessation, sleep issues, and bipolar disorder. Some off-label uses of the drug may be effective; however, the drug is also associated with suicidal acts and violent deaths.[12] Likewise, misuse of the opioid OxyContin has been widely reported by the media over the past several years. Sales of this drug rose almost six-fold from 1997 to 2005,[13] a period when recreational use of this addictive heroin-like drug became a societal problem. Our system helps detect unusual patterns and potential safety risks of drugs.

I believe all physicians entering medicine today need to think carefully about how to position themselves in a network of knowledge sharing and learning. Too much is in a state of flux for us to be successful as fiercely independent lone rangers. We need to expect that our ways of practicing medicine will be constantly challenged. We need to be prepared to work with our patients, who may come armed with marketing information, in order to arrive at the best evidence-based treatment course. We need to abandon practices when new knowledge and better approaches become available. And, we need to make decisions to not use new, often more expensive, approaches, if the evidence does not support that they will be better for our patient.

Practicing According to the Evidence Does Not Mean Giving Up Clinical Judgment

Evidence-based practice (EBP) does have detractors. Clinicians fear that it will take away their autonomy and that suggested guidelines will be turned into regulations that must be followed in any given case.[14] The term "cookbook medicine" is sometimes mentioned.[15] Critics also feel that such an approach to medicine denigrates it from a profession to something that can be done by lower-paid, less-skilled technicians.[16] There are also some philosophers of science who dispute the notion of science being objective and value-free, and criticize EBP on these grounds. This creates debates about the relative importance of clinical experience and the scientific basis of medicine. I believe this is a silly discussion since clearly both are important, as I have been discussing throughout the book. For physicians, the key question is how to become better and better clinicians, which includes incorporating new scientific knowledge into our practices.

Defenders state that EBP should never substitute for a doctor's experience and judgment in the face of a given case; rather, it should be a firm foundation to bolster, guide, and support a physician in his or her choice of action. EBP should not mean that doctors are automatons just thoughtlessly following a flowchart when treating patients. In SCPMG, doctors craft the guidelines. EBP-based guidelines incorporate the most efficacious, safe, and appropriate treatments and medicines for patients. But we also recognize that each patient is unique. In fact much of today's evidence is shining systematic light on the fact that different procedures should be applied toward patients with different risk factors. Increasingly, the scientific evidence is examining individual differences such as in genetic structure—and uncovering associated differences in efficacious treatment paths. One can't get much more individualized than that.

Doctors in the US have not enthusiastically embraced EBP. In fact, adoption of evidence-based practice has been described as modest.[17] This is changing. Recent legislation, including the 2010 Affordable Care Act (ACA) and the American Recovery and Reinvestment Act (ARRA) of 2009 both include provisions that will serve to further advance EBP. ARRA will authorize over one billion dollars in comparative effectiveness research. The ACA will establish the non-profit Patient-Centered Outcomes Research Institute.[18] These will certainly contribute to an increase in EBP. Following best practice as advocated in the literature is already an important defensive practice that can support a doctor's course of action in court. It will rapidly be tied to quality measures that impact reimbursements. It's coming. We need to be ready for it by making sure we're linked to knowledge. We need to make sure that we physicians define the implications of the evidence base. And we need to make sure this is done in a way that we can address the requirements of individual patients. We can't do it alone. We need to band together and work with other stakeholders to make sure this happens.

Continuing Medical Education

Part of the professionalism of being a physician is continuous learning. There is a real pride in keeping oneself up to date as a doctor. I always feel energized after attending a conference or lecture. I have walked away with new, up-to-date information–or confirmation that I am doing the right thing for my patients. This meshes neatly with the philosophy behind EBP, which requires an ongoing learning process that continues for the entire career of a physician. A doctor will always be discovering new procedures and ways of more effectively practicing medicine. [19]

Most states in the US require continuing medical education (CME) for licensure reregistration. For example, MDs in California have to complete fifty CME credits every two years, and doctors in Texas have to complete twenty-four credits per year. Some states also mandate specific content: Connecticut, for example, requires coursework in infectious disease, risk management, sexual assault, domestic violence, and cultural competence.[20] Physicians need a strategy for keeping up with these requirements.

SCPMG actively helps our physicians with the recertification process, and more generally, makes it easy and convenient for them to get their CME credits and stay up to date in their knowledge base. We produce a primer with all the latest information and knowledge needed for doctors undergoing the recertification process. The primer is tied into structured symposia that run over three weeks.

More generally, 10 percent of a SCPMG physician's time is set aside for education–that works out to half a day of education time every week plus one week of educational leave every year. Our various specialty groups use regular CME-approved webinars to explore different issues in the practice. They assemble experts in the field to discuss innovative practices and new knowledge, and provide mechanisms for our physicians to share best practices. SCPMG physicians can take very inexpensive CME courses from us. These are ways we help doctors meet the prodigious learning challenge. Physicians make their own clinical decisions, but their continual exposure to and discussion of the evidence through CME courses leads to a great deal of convergence on effective approaches. A dedication to continuing education is not just lip service; it's a clear expectation of our doctors.

Although there has been an increase in regulation pertaining to whether and how pharmaceutical companies can fund CME, lots of education and continuing education events are still funded by big pharma.[21] Pharmaceutical company support for CME has declined since 2008, but there is still a great deal of controversy over whether doctors can objectively detach outside company funding for CME from any sort of favoritism in prescribing medication. We at SCPMG have tried to avoid this problem by developing our own content based on the literature, and delivering it without the biases of corporate interest.

There are a myriad of ways for all physicians, whether in a large system or not, to take part in continuing education. Groups like the American Medical Association (AMA) offer activities for credit. Online courses are offered by the *Journal of the AMA* for members and subscribers; in the UK, *BMJ* (formerly *British Medical Journal*) also offers online courses that are accredited by many bodies. There are traditional lecture-like presentations, conferences, and symposia, as well as more interactive live events, like workshops and programs that specifically focus on practice-enabling strategies and reinforcing methods.[22] There is a large industry devoted to producing these events.[23] So with a forest of possible ways to get CME, it comes down to being the responsibility of each individual person taking charge of his or her own continuing medical education.[24]

In continuing their education, physicians benefit from being part of rich learning networks. In the attitudes toward CME, and in determining whether a doctor adopts evidence-based practices, the influence of professional colleagues is critical. If the colleagues we interact with on a face-to-face basis are seekers and advocates of evidence-based practice, then it's more likely we will be as well. Active communities of practice are crucial components in our professional lives as doctors to share knowledge and to grow as professionals. Indeed, the generous exposure to shared learning with my colleagues is one reason I stayed in SCPMG for over three decades. Whether this is through a large system or some other form of collegial network is not the point. The point is that in today's world, we can't do this without the network.

CME at the Point of Care

Another practice, which is increasingly possible and that we are finding to be quite effective, we call "CME at the point of care."[25] More broadly, this is referred to as clinical decision support (CDS). When you have an electronic medical record in every examining room, why not make it easy to deliver the most up-to-date information right then and there? Leverage the awesome power of the IT system and make it easier for the doctor at the same time.

As an example, in 2009, the American College of Obstetrics and Gynecologists revised its Pap smear screening guidelines (for women over thirty with a negative HPV/not at higher-risk for cervical cancer) from each year to every three years. Other outside agencies and quality rating organizations have since converged on similar guidelines. How can we make sure that every physician knows about this relatively new guideline? Make it as obvious as possible. Make sure that it's right there when a doctor opens the woman's electronic medical record. This is an example of how we disseminate new knowledge in the form of new procedures, protocols, and technologies. We do not constrain the physician's decision, but we draw attention to the change in guidelines.

In addition, when something major is changing, SCPMG immediately sends out Rapid Response Statement e-mails to affected doctors. The Rapid Response Statement is just-in-time delivery of information. It tells doctors what is happening, what it means, and suggests how to deal with affected patients. To show the speed with which change and adjustment is required, recently in just a two-week period the FDA issued guidance on four drugs: 1) warning that finasteride, although efficacious in treating prostate cancer in general, is possibly linked to more aggressive, high-risk prostate cancer, 2) limiting the recommended dose of simvastatin because of possible muscle injury, 3) linking Actos to bladder cancer when used in diabetics, and 4) no longer recommending Avastin for metastatic breast cancer because of significant side effects and no evidence that it improves mortality. We passed this guidance on to all our physicians. At about the same time, new information came out about the efficacy of CT scanning for lung cancer detection. Even though this new evidence suggests that these scans can detect lung cancer, before we make the leap to screen everyone, our physicians are further assessing the data and making a careful determination of whether to change our guidelines.

Working with Dr. Joanne Schottinger and her Clinical Practice Guideline Group, our physician leaders shape the content of the e-mail blasts about changes in FDA guidance about a drug, and help determine the action that is required to reach affected patients. We determine how best to work with people currently on the drug. We often mobilize care managers to work with our patients, thus supporting the doctor in rapidly responding to this new information. Such rapid implementation of change, including the outreach to all affected patients, would not be possible if our health system were not staffed and designed for the detection and implementation of knowledge—and, to support our physicians in responding. Ultimately our physicians write the changes to practice guidelines that result from this new information.

Many health systems, healthcare IT organizations and vendors are developing clinical decision making support systems for specific high-volume diseases and/or to detect and alert physicians to drug interactions. For example, HealthPartners and GroupHealth in Minnesota have developed and tested a "Diabetes Wizard" as part of the National Institutes of Health funding of clinical trials to improve diabetes care.[26] The AT&T Healthcare Community Online Physician Portal positions itself as almost a one-stop shop for health IT applications and solutions for physicians.[27] Isabel Healthcare offers "Isabel," a diagnosis checklist, directly to physicians; its subscription rates range from $250 to $375 annually, putting this kind of web-based decision support within range even of individual practitioners.[28] In today's world of rapid development of healthcare knowledge and fast-paced medical care delivery, it's essential that physicians have access to high-quality, evidence-based decision support.

Expect to Be Lifelong Learners

Physicians are professionals whose calling demands continuous, lifelong learning. What we have learned from evidence-based practice yesterday may be superseded by new medical discoveries or technical innovations tomorrow. For the sake of our patients, our society, and ourselves, we doctors must keep up with new knowledge and incorporate it to change how we practice medicine. Otherwise we are dinosaurs who can do more harm than good in our ignorance, consuming resources without delivering the needed value.

Here again, this is a great time to be a physician. Rapidly advancing access to electronic applications and information sources facilitates continuous learning. This is especially true if physicians form rich networks for sharing knowledge and contributing to the learning of the profession. Such communities of practice can have significant positive impact on the health status of our patients and the populations we serve.

Trend	Implications for Physicians	Am I effectively dealing with this trend now?
Dizzying Increase in Amount and Rate of Growth of Medical Knowledge		
	1. Physicians will have strategies to keep current with latest evidence-based information, technology and techniques. 2. Doctors can effectively connect to a knowledge support network that interprets and distills research for and with its members. 3. Sharing and interpretation of new trends and knowledge among fellow physicians is the most powerful dissemination approach. 4. Physicians work to translate the latest findings into practice guidelines.	
Outside Influences on Our Medical Practice		
	1. Many patients request specific drugs/procedures because of pharmaceutical company advertising. 2. Doctors, not insurance companies, should prescribe drugs.	
Continuous, Lifelong Learning		
	1. Recertification and CME credits can be met in a myriad of ways. 2. Learning networks and communities of practice are crucial in our professional lives. 3. Clinical decision support allows for "CME at the point of care."	

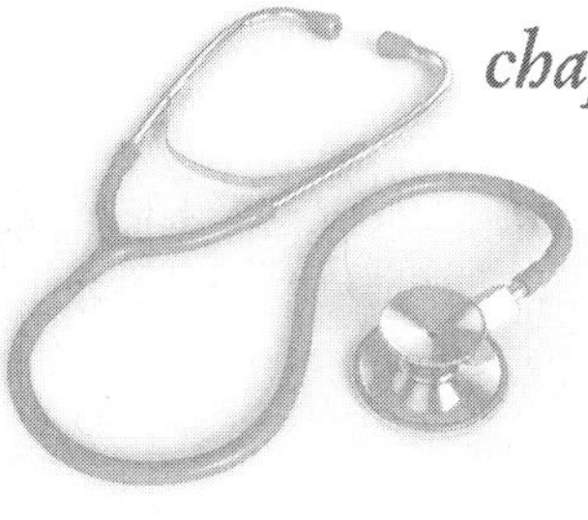

chapter seven

Innovation and Improvement

The ability to generate ongoing creative solutions is essential in business today. Yet the organization of healthcare has only recently begun to change to reflect the new realities. How much innovation and improvement does it take to reverse the frankly unsustainable healthcare-related cost increases that many Americans struggle with daily? A lot! And that's why we physicians need to decide that we will be part of the process, so that we build a more viable healthcare system for the future. We can make a big difference to the health of our patients and the population as a whole if we contribute to the innovation that is required. And, I believe, we will have immensely more satisfying practices as a result.

Organizations such as the Institute for Healthcare Improvement (IHI) have played an important role. They have made healthcare systems aware of the need to incorporate evidence into healthcare practices and processes, to systematically improve processes, and to innovate. They have developed courses and learning communities in these areas that have infused a great deal of knowledge into the healthcare community. They build on quality and process improvement methodologies that have radically increased the efficiency and effectiveness of processes in other sectors of our economy. Indeed, our efforts at Kaiser Permanente have drawn on the methodologies IHI has developed. In this book, I mention many other healthcare systems that have introduced innovative approaches and built improvement into the way they operate. These include Intermountain Healthcare, the Cleveland Clinic, HealthCare Partners, Montefiore, Fairview, Geisinger, and the Veteran's Administration Healthcare System, to name just a few. For these organizations, innovation and improvement have become a way of life, part of an ongoing journey to develop sustainable models of healthcare delivery in today's demanding environment.

Physicians are accustomed to adopting new and innovative drugs, devices, diagnostic and treatment technologies, and procedures. Examples that we have incorporated into our work are robotics, minimally invasive surgery, cytology testing, genetic screenings, and biologics. These new products and innovations increase our clinical capabilities but leave our patterns of practice fundamentally unchanged. They are often expensive. Societies then face even greater challenges to secure the resources to take advantage of these wondrous new therapeutic approaches.

Physicians also need to play our part in generating innovative approaches to increase value so that high-quality healthcare can be sustainably delivered. Otherwise the forces of change will continue to drag us along toward rationing, cost shifting, and draconian limits on healthcare spending. This will result in increasing inequities in the provision of healthcare to the population we serve. We will see ourselves as victims of decisions that limit our ability to deliver on the promise of modern healthcare. We can't expect others to change around us and believe we will be left alone to practice medicine in our comfort zones.

Physicians also need to play our part in generating innovative approaches to increase value so that high-quality healthcare can be sustainably delivered. Otherwise the forces of change will continue to drag us along toward rationing, cost shifting, and draconian limits on healthcare spending.

Value is defined as "health outcomes achieved per dollar spent."[1] It is achieved by increasing the ratio of the quality of services that are delivered and outcomes achieved to the resources that are consumed in the process. In pursuing value, healthcare will follow in the footsteps of other sectors such as telecommunications, media, and financial services. These have combined new technology, lean operations, customer focus, and new ways of organizing and providing service. The result has been convenient, high-quality, affordable services and products that were unimaginable just decades ago. Movies can be streamed into your house less expensively than a trip to a movie theater, and you have the comfort and convenience of watching from home. You can now make a free, high-quality Internet phone call to anywhere in the world, or hold a videoconference with participants on every continent. You can buy and sell securities from the convenience of your home or office, see models and growth projections for your portfolio online, and receive high-quality information and advice about how to weather the current financial upheaval. You can do research on most topics online for very little expense rather than going to libraries or buying books or journals. These disruptive changes have enabled new forms of organization and new business models and at the same time have ended many businesses that at one time were highly successful (think of Circuit City, Borders Books, or Sun Microsystems).

We're already seeing innovations that augur great change in the way healthcare is delivered. Retail health providers such as MinuteClinics are taking primary care to the patient's everyday haunts. Home monitoring and remote monitoring, secure e-mailing to your physician, and telemedicine have arrived. These are quickly freeing patients and physicians from their dependence on the cycle of periodic and emergency visits to healthcare facilities, and moving to just-in-time delivery of care. Life-cycle care is challenging the transactional, episodic, and uncoordinated manner in which various healthcare providers have treated people with chronic conditions. The EMR is enabling patients to easily cross state and national boundaries to get care from providers with the best value. And with increased reporting of outcomes and cost information, patients are rapidly climbing into the driver's seat seeking the best care for the dollar spent.

Increasing value has been our mantra for the past eight years at SCPMG, and we've approached this by seeking innovative ways to increase the health status of our member population and achieve operational efficiencies. In 1960, Sidney Garfield, MD, Kaiser Permanente's innovative co-founder, counseled that healthcare was facing a new frontier. Rather than simply building hospitals and clinics to treat illness, he believed it was time to build a healthcare system "for health."[2] We've been heeding his advice. Many of our innovations are geared to keep people healthy, delaying the onset and progression of chronic disease, keeping people from having acute flare-ups along with their damaging side effects, increasing patient safety, reduce the need for hospitalization, and helping people take control and manage their own health.

I believe that building a system for health is the challenge facing all of medicine. It is a particular challenge for physicians, as most of us have been socialized to think of ourselves as having a role to cure and treat, rather than to prevent. Curing and treating will always remain immensely important, and indeed are central to healthcare built for wellness. The role of the physician remains pivotal. But we cannot continue to take a narrow view of our accountabilities.

Our bet at SCPMG is that increasing quality of care and outcomes goes hand in hand with keeping people well and lowering costs. Healthcare dollars saved by avoiding unnecessary treatment can fund investments needed to keep people well. This will make the healthcare dollar go further in treating those who, despite our best efforts or due to the unalterable progression of time and aging, need to be treated for any number of serious conditions. Of course disease and the deterioration of the body cannot be fully prevented. But delaying onset and maintaining health to the extent possible will definitely increase value to individuals and society in terms of both outcomes and costs.

Why wait for elderly patients to take a fall and fracture a hip before diagnosing osteoporosis and starting treatment? Shouldn't we give as much importance to avoiding strokes and heart attacks by vigilantly keeping hypertension under control as we do to providing heroic measures with thrombolytics when they do occur? As pediatricians, we can only do so much medically to start children on the road to health. Wouldn't we be better off if our efforts were supplemented by the health education families need to foster healthy lifestyles and get their kids off the couch and their hands out of the cookie jar? These are some of the many areas where we are developing new practices.

A Vision

Ten years ago, I sat in Paul's Café in Tarzana, California with Drs. Paul Minardi and Michael Kanter (later to become the regional medical director of Operations and regional medical director of Quality and Clinical Analysis, respectively) and we contemplated what medicine could be if we built a system for health and used all the resources at our disposal to make our population of patients as healthy as they could possibly be. It was a lofty vision—but the hard work hadn't begun. Even though KP has been a leader in prevention efforts from its beginning, we knew it would take new ways of thinking, a great deal of change, and the introduction of innovative approaches. Prevention has been underfunded and understaffed in our society, and as a result, we've ended up with a system that focuses almost exclusively on treatment. Primary care physicians have struggled with an impossible load on their shoulders in trying to do prevention well. We felt we needed to change that.

Many, but not all, SCPMG physicians have reacted favorably to this vision. We know that in any organization there will be some who will welcome the chance to innovate. The largest percent will go along with change if it can be shown to make a difference in performance. And there's another group who will resist change, period. We've made it easy for the group of innovators to surface and try things out. We've thrown out challenges to the system, encouraged new practices and provided resources for pilots. And when results are demonstrated, we've worked to scale up the changes and support broader dissemination. Hundreds of change champions and innovators have played a role in building a system focused on value.

We are a long way from the finish line. In fact, we at SCPMG are still in the early stages of the journey. Each step along the way relies on many physicians and others in the system coming up with and championing new approaches to the way we work and on the hard work of testing, refining, and dissemination. Because we've insisted that all innovative approaches use resources wisely to continuously raise the bar on quality of care, improved outcomes, and improved health status, our physicians have gradually moved from being skeptics to being proud of what we're accomplishing. Physicians respond to statistically accurate data. We've used measurement and evaluation to test the value of new approaches, and we have continually refined our approaches to ensure that we are positively impacting value.

We know we can't keep raising prices, so we're always asking some important questions. Where can we free up resources from the unimportant or unnecessary to direct them to the reason we're all here? What evidence is there that something really makes a difference? If there isn't any, let's not do it. Pap smear screening is an example. In 2006, the standard of care was for women to receive yearly Pap smears. With the advent of HPV testing, evidence pointed toward shifting to less frequent Pap smear testing. The NCQA measures for quality, as well as the guidelines of the American Cancer Society (ACS) and the American Congress of Obstetricians and Gynecologists (ACOG), support three-year intervals for women over the age of thirty with prior normal exams. Now at KPSC, 93 percent of our women receive Pap smears according to our new guidelines, compared to 58 percent five years ago. At the same time, more women are being screened, and we are doing better at early cervical cancer detection. From 2006 to 2008, we increased our cervical cancer screening rate from 79 percent to 87 percent of the targeted population. We said we were moving away from "over-Pap-ulation,"

Two Views of Innovation

Dr. Todd Sachs, Chief of Surgery for West Los Angeles

"Innovation has been an emphasis at SCPMG. This includes areas like HealthConnect and medical innovations like robotic surgery. We put a clinical acumen into our innovation to make sure we're using and building evidence. We get a lot of help from the organization to make sure we don't jump on the bandwagon of the newfangled toy. We want to make sure there is real merit and value added when we adopt something new. To me that is very important. We have teams that look at what is the best practice. What new drugs, devices, and procedures make a difference?"

Dr. Brian Nguyen, Physician Director of Clinical Strategic Goals Optimization

"We have to innovate to survive. Patients are changing, practices are changing and technology is changing. Front-line physicians are the best people to innovate. They see and understand the need. I'm fortunate to practice medicine where I have the ability to innovate. With six thousand physicians you could feel like you are a small drop in the sea. The areas that do this well have open communication and clear channels to bring ideas to physician leaders. There are channels to get attention and support from the administration to try out new ideas."

and the shift required widespread education and acceptance by all our physicians. When is the most expensive approach well worth the cost because it delivers better outcomes, and when is it just plain more expensive? Many of our ophthalmologists were using the drug Lucentis to treat wet age-related macular degeneration. Evidence showed that it was no more efficacious than the existing drug Avastin, but was more expensive. So we changed our prescription recommendations and freed up resources for other purposes. Presently we're working on how best to integrate the newly releasted drug Eylea into our treatment recommendations.

Where should we expend more resources that will raise the health status of our patients and lead to less demand on our acute care systems? Vaccines administered to prevent cervical cancer and shingles and fecal immunochemical testing for colon cancer result in higher costs, but better quality. Where can we achieve greater impact by greater teamwork and coordination? Team-based care for geriatrics and palliation is essential. And what kind of workflows and organizing approaches will make all these things happen? Redesigning message management and in-basket management when using an electronic medical record is necessary to support physicians. Developing systems and workflows to coordinate complex processes such as post-hospital discharge can result in greater efficiency and effectiveness.

By continually asking these questions, challenging our physicians to achieve world-class performance, and by providing the support and resources to make change, we have seen more and more physician innovators step forward and change the nature of how we do work. Our integrated system has been fortunate to have an extremely gifted set of administrators and expert staff in our medical group, as well as in the Kaiser Foundation Hospitals and Health Plan organizations, who have teamed up with our physicians in resetting how we think about, organize, and carry out healthcare.

Four areas where we have focused our innovation to create what I believe to be the conditions for sustaining effective healthcare in the future are:

1) The Complete Care model builds in proactive touch points with our members, segments our population, and develops approaches to ensure that the healthcare needs of each segment are met.

2) We are developing effective multidisciplinary processes that cut across the lifecycle of disease.

3) We are building a learning system to continuously improve our clinical and operational processes.

4) We are empowering patients to take responsibility for their health.

These areas of needed change are not unique to large integrated healthcare systems like Kaiser Permanente. I would argue that they are integral to any true healthcare reform that enhances the value of healthcare. They have profound implications for how we practice medicine.

Complete Care

A problem faced by our country is: how does our healthcare system turn the dial to place a greater focus toward proactively keeping our population well rather than continuing to spend more and more resources responding to illness? How do we move toward outcomes-driven healthcare? These are the same puzzles we set out to solve at SCPMG, and we believe we are gradually putting many of the pieces into place. We call our approach "Complete Care," because we've focused on improved outcomes and total health of our population of members. And to do this we've essentially had to invent new approaches to reach out to over three million members with very diverse healthcare needs. My colleagues Dr. Michael Kanter and Dr. Paul Minardi have masterminded these approaches and assembled a tremendous team to help design, implement, and continuously improve them. They have encouraged innovative approaches throughout the system, ensured assessment of impact on outcomes and efficiency, and supported broad dissemination of effective approaches.

Proactive Care. A problem we set out to solve was how to proactively reach millions of members to make sure that they receive the care appropriate to their needs. We wanted to deal with the whole person, not just with presenting symptoms or current crises. Our intent is to make our members' experiences seamless across all their healthcare needs, from ambulatory care, including wellness and prevention, to urgent and emergency care, acute illness, chronic disease treatment, and end-of-life care.

SCPMG has crafted organizational approaches for proactive identification and filling of care gaps among a population of members, some of whom do not regularly come to see us, to find out what they should be doing to maintain their health and/or keep their conditions under control. The value we derive from registries has been increased by identifying key segments of our population with particular disease states or treatment conditions. These registries allow us to reach out to individual patients in these segments to make sure they are on an appropriate treatment course. We are able to track certain populations of patients to prevent severe medical complications such as smokers over age sixty who have a higher incidence of aortic aneurysm. By researching best practices, we have developed approaches to patient resources and education that are integrated into our Complete Care approach. And we have redesigned our workflows to get our many healthcare professionals and staff more directly involved in improving our members' health. These approaches and the many others we have put in place have required a great deal of innovation throughout all areas of our organization, our business model, and our workflows.

The vision of complete care couldn't be achieved merely by asking physicians to practice differently, worry about more things, and take on additional coordination responsibilities. Physicians are already overloaded. Providing complete care for our members required changes in the systems in which we operate. We had to develop new workflows, teams, roles, and information systems to allow people across many professional groups and specialties to focus on the patient, while using standard and predictable processes that enable us all to work together as one big virtual team.

Various physician and non-physician leaders in our system have accepted this challenge and have risen to the occasion to innovate. They have crafted and piloted fundamental changes to the more fragmented, episodic, and narrow conception of healthcare that has permeated Western medicine. We've had a talented group of programmers who have built new capabilities onto the core platform of our EMR. We need new and advanced tools that allow our physicians and other members of the team to do their jobs in new ways. The vast amount of information that is now available has been parceled into applications tailored to the immediate work needs of physicians, nurses, medical assistants, pharmacists, nutritionists, and others who deal with the patient.

With our new systems, for example, our physicians have ready access to patients' pharmacy histories and can detect non-compliance. In KPSC's integrated medical adherence program, physicians can see flags about non-adherence and about possible drug safety issues such as excessive bleeding when patients on anticoagulants are concurrently taking NSAIDS. Pharmacists and care managers can reach out to patients who are non-compliant and/or in danger from drug interactions. Patients receive automated refill reminders and get pharmaceutical counseling regarding side effects and dosing from pharmacists who are knowledgeable about their medical history.

The systems also enable medical assistants or call center agents to contact patients in advance of a scheduled appointment to make sure that they arrive with all the needed tests having been completed. This saves extra appointments and the dissatisfaction that occurs when the physician can't complete an assessment because of insufficient or delayed data. Outreach and care managers can ensure that chronically ill patients receive care when needed rather than at conventionally accepted intervals. A diabetic whose HbA1c demonstrates poor control will benefit from a switch to insulin from their oral medication and should not wait. Reminders about physicians' orders can be communicated by electronic alerts to the patient, thus increasing the likelihood of compliance.

Everyone's job has changed. The whole team has information to deliver patient-focused care. Our Proactive Office Support system makes sure that our back office staff assists in carrying out the needed management of in-basket data and timely message management. In addition, nurses support physicians in identifying care gaps in their patient panels. I previously described the Proactive Office Encounter (POE), the set of standard workflows and processes to make sure that when patients come in to the system for a primary or specialty visit, test, or to pick up medications, the people they deal with alert them to needed prevention tests or care gaps. Similarly, the Proactive Inpatient Encounter has been designed to efficiently and reliably address pre-hospitalization, admission and inpatient experiences and discharge/post-hospitalization care needs. These are standard processes that increase the responsibility of everyone who has a touch point with the patient for ensuring that all care processes are carried out. We also use this approach in the emergency room.

Segmentation. The healthcare of the majority of our patients is managed and monitored by a primary care physician and the office team through a standard panel management process. In our increasingly sophisticated complete care approach, automated electronic tools detect and flag abnormal results that are followed up on by the front-line staff. An abnormal PSA, potassium, creatinine, or Pap smear does not go unnoticed.

Many patients with chronic conditions and multiple morbidities require more care touches. We have identified different segments, or sub-populations, that require more continuous care and more active management of that care. Care managers proactively review the care of the population of those with COPD, diabetes, and other chronic illnesses against practice guidelines. They identify where there are care gaps and/or uncontrolled symptoms and initiate action. A case management team deals with patients with complex conditions such as ESRD, HIV, CHF, and Hepatitis C. A patient's care team is recomposed as the patient moves through various stages of the disease, and different kinds of touch points are established. And we have created a safety net of a small centralized team that monitors small groups of patients at high outpatient risk who might otherwise fall through the cracks.

We've developed this segmentation approach and organized to systematically reach out to our diverse member sub-populations to make sure their care needs are met appropriately. Our purpose is to keep each member as close as possible to the healthy end of the life cycle continuum.

Integrating Care Along the Lifecycle of Disease

In the US, over 75 percent of our healthcare dollars go toward care for the chronically ill.[3] The annual cost of chronic disease in the US, including healthcare expenses, lost income, and lost productivity, is estimated to be over one trillion dollars.[4] By 2020, an estimated 157 million people will have at least one chronic condition, and spending for chronic conditions will account for 80 percent of all healthcare spending.[5] A major cause is lifestyle, and any chronic disease program has to start with that, preferably well before the onset of disease. Yet we know that for many, the onset of disease will come and that these patients will suffer and have a greatly degraded quality of life as they go through the various stages of the disease. Innovative approaches to dealing with prevention and lifecycle treatment of chronic conditions is becoming a major focus throughout the US. This is definitely an area of emphasis at KPSC.

Healthy Bones. Our Healthy Bones Model of Care is an example of an innovative approach to chronic illness that arose from the vision of Dr. Richard Dell, an orthopedic surgeon from Downey Medical Center, who felt that we could greatly reduce the incidence of osteoporosis and fragility fractures caused by osteoporosis in our population. A multidisciplinary team developed what has turned into our "Healthy Bones" program. It has greatly expanded preventive screening as well as increased the treatment for osteoporosis, and decreased the incidence of hip fractures.[6] The team includes people from orthopedics, physical therapy, endocrinology, rheumatology, radiology, family medicine, internal medicine, nephrology, and pharmacy, as well as care managers, and is underpinned by the skills of our IT department. Although it started small in one medical center, the clear results have led to an expansion of the program to all medical centers.

The EMR is used to identify and initiate outreach by care managers to people in our target groups, which includes women over sixty-five, men over seventy, and those with personal histories of fracture or related health problems. DXA scans and FRAX calculations are interpreted immediately. Where indicated, we then walk patients to "Just in Time" clinics, which are located in each medical center. At the clinic, care managers thoroughly discuss the scan results with the patient. Individualized plans are developed, which may include treatment with bisphosphonates or other anti-osteoporosis treatments such as vitamin and mineral supplementation, lifestyle and safety interventions, and fall assessment. We aim for this clinic to be a one-stop shop for our osteoporotic patients. Evidence-based care management guidelines have been created, patients are entered into registries, and care managers identify care gaps and deficiencies. Our program is now rated number one in the nation by HEDIS. Because of our population-wide approach to proactively and automatically detecting those at risk and initiating screening and treatment, we have also reduced traditional ethnic disparities in medical treatment for osteoporosis.[7] The Healthy Bones program serves as a model for the development of similar programs throughout the Kaiser Permanente national program. In addition, the Healthy Bones Model of Care is gaining both national and international recognition as a comprehensive and effective approach to the prevention and management of osteoporosis.

Healthy Bones Model of Care and Osteoporosis

The Need:

- Twenty-four percent of people with hip fractures die within a year of the fracture
- Hip fractures account for approximately 63 percent of all cost of fragility fractures
- Each hip fracture costs approximately $37,000 to treat

The Healthy Bones Program Elements:

- Proactive screening of at-risk members and immediate treatment with medicine, exercise, dietary, and safety recommendations
- Care managers, multidisciplinary team, and Just-in-Time Clinics for same day screening and commencement of treatment
- All of KPSC's medical centers have been involved with Healthy Bones since 2002
- Between 2002 and 2009, KPSC's annual number of DXA scans increased 474 percent, from 21,557 to 123,664[8]

The Results:

- Approximately 1,069 fractures were prevented by this program in 2009
- Approximate savings: 257 lives and roughly $39.5 million
- By 2010, KPSC saw over a 45 percent reduction in the number of hip fractures, based on comparison to what would be expected using projected data from 2000.
- KPSC ranked number one in the country for its osteoporosis program in 2006 and every year thereafter by HEDIS.

Arthritis and Healthy Joints. The importance of managing the full disease cycle of arthritis patients was identified by Dr. Tad Funahashi, the regional chief of Orthopedic Surgery. Our improvement of the total joint process at KPSC primarily deals with an episode of care—joint replacement surgery—that has to fit into a larger care pathway. We realized that more significant arthritis care can and should be done before resorting to surgery, in order to optimize the patient's condition and to delay surgery as long as possible. A care pathway was created by an interdisciplinary team and is coordinated by orthopedic surgeons and care managers. A specific protocol is created when the patient experiences the first episode of severe joint pain. It focuses on nutrition, weight loss, exercise, and medication management, including arthritis medication and joint pain treatment. This care pathway prevents the patient from going to the stage of total joint replacement earlier than necessary. This pilot program is being tested at our Orange County Medical Center and eventually, if proven to be efficacious, will be transferred throughout our organization.

Back Pain. Between 60 and 80 percent of the population will suffer from debilitating lower back pain during their lifetime. It is a leading cause for absence from work and accounted for eighty-three million sick days in the US in 1996.[9] It's a condition that is associated with great human suffering and cost to our society. Medical systems have had a fragmented approach to deal with lower back pain. Different care pathways are likely to be recommended depending on whether the patient sees a primary care physician, goes to an emergency room or an urgent care, or sees an orthopedist, a neurologist, or a physiatrist. To reduce this variation and make sure our patients get on an optimal care pathway very quickly, we have developed a streamlined care process for lower back pain patients. Our goal is to quickly start them on a therapeutic regimen, achieve a more timely reduction in pain, where possible prevent the condition from becoming chronic, and to reduce the incidence of back surgery and unnecessary exposure to radiation from CT and MRI scans.

Dr. Kim Thai, regional chief of Physical Medicine & Rehabilitation and our lead physician for Acute Back Pain Management, was one of the physicians I met with in my office to talk about this problem. The pilot program at our Foothill/Pasadena clinic is now being rolled out to all our regional medical centers. The approach is simple: we put resources up front for the patient. When a patient contacts our call center about lower back pain, that call is directly transferred to the back pain clinic without the patient having to make another call. Patients meet jointly with a physical medicine doctor and a physical therapist on the same day they call or the following day. Together they create a plan of care, which may include a same-day appointment with physical therapy.

The back pain clinic avoids the escalation of symptoms that would occur if a patient had to go through a series of different office visits to get to the point of beginning a treatment plan. Initial findings show that people treated this way average four visits to the clinic before declaring that their pain has subsided. The majority of the lower back patients in the pilot who reported the most severe pain reported a measurable decrease in pain on the Modified Oswestry Disability Index (MODI) after just one treatment. I believe this program, when adopted at all our medical centers, will truly afford profound relief to our KPSC patients who suffer from this common condition.

These examples all point to the power of taking an interdisciplinary approach to defining the most effective care pathway for complex conditions that require multiple treatment modalities. They also demonstrate the power of taking a preventive approach to reduce the trauma to the patient from aggressive treatment that might be avoided or delayed. SCPMG physicians have led the interdisciplinary teams that have generated these approaches, and our regional chiefs of service and the chiefs in each medical center work closely with our different physician specialties, care managers, pharmacists, and others to implement them in a way that fits each local unit.

Health systems all over the world are working to optimize care pathways. At SCPMG, we still have many more opportunities to optimize care pathways and achieve better outcomes with less cost and less suffering. We have come to appreciate that we cannot simply systematize what we are already doing. Rather, to change outcomes requires building on evidence and innovating. It is our responsibility as physicians to make sure that that innovation is guided by sound medical knowledge and that the new pathways lead to high-quality outcomes and enhance the value that we deliver to our patients and to society.

Building an Ongoing Learning System for Clinical and Operational Improvement

Building heath systems that are guided by evidence is a national challenge. The variation in practice across our country and among physicians leads to unnecessary cost and uneven outcomes.[10] Yet we continue to see such variation, even as information about the efficacy of various practices proliferates, as do the tools and resources to provide the evidence to physicians. I don't believe this extreme variation in application of evidence and in outcomes can or should continue.

Evidence-based medicine is clearly not a concept we came up with at Kaiser Permanente, but it is one that we've been concerned about for decades. Evidence underpins all of our innovation at SCPMG, including clinical innovation, change in delivery systems, service systems, and organizational approaches. We've developed approaches that we believe have moved us much closer to being an evidence-based system. These approaches enable our physicians to interpret and adapt to a rapidly changing evidence base. The challenge we face is to develop approaches that involve physician leadership and involvement so that a staff of six thousand physicians in many specialty areas, trained in many different medical schools and distributed over many thousands of square miles, are guided by up-to-date evidence. To address this challenge, we have developed approaches to build learning into how we operate.

In chapter six, I described some of the systematic approaches we have developed over the years to build an evidence-based learning system. I emphasized the importance of physician leadership and involvement in scrutinizing and interpreting the data and translating evidence into practice guidelines and tools. I also emphasized providing physicians with resources and support to enable them to quickly and easily incorporate new evidence into their busy practices. And in chapter eight I will discuss the role of both disciplinary and multidisciplinary teams in crafting and executing these learning approaches.

Learning Across the Region. These three principles—physician leadership, multidisciplinary teams, and providing physicians with resources and support to learn–come together in such bodies as our Drug Utilization Action Team (DUAT) that was described in chapter five, and our Radiology Utilization Action Team (RUAT), which will be more fully described in the next chapter. These are multidisciplinary, physician-led bodies, composed from across the region. They play the very critical function of reviewing the research evidence in the context of the goals and vision of KPSC, translating it into recommended practice, and defining appropriate metrics. Similarly composed teams deal with the articulation of our various chronic disease pathways and process improvement initiatives, and with many other issues that require care coordination across our diverse providers.

Our radiologists, pharmacists and clinical researchers continually scan the literature and organize the evidence regarding drug and x-ray use. SCPMG clinical leaders are gathering evidence as well, and they debate the literature and work together to translate these into guidelines, decision support, processes and pathways, and communications to keep our physicians up to date and aide them in their own professional task of continuous learning (see chapter six for a description of how this occurs).

You're probably thinking that this approach is easy to do in a big integrated system with sufficient resources. But is this possible in the world of private practice, where there are small physician groups and many different independent provider organizations that have to coordinate to deliver healthcare and where insurance companies are trying to extract every dollar possible from healthcare premiums? Of course it is true that our size and formal structure help. But this hasn't been easy even for us, and it has involved persistence and hard work across many different stakeholders. We have had to rethink the assumptions that were built into our highly departmentalized and segmented organization. Everyone wanted to control things and didn't want to work together. Most physicians thought theirs was the best practice. And we had to create and implement new organizational approaches to get people to sit down and learn from each other.

If we are to deliver greater value for healthcare dollars, that same rethinking and inventing of new ways to learn and improve will have to characterize all healthcare systems, whether formally integrated or not. I've mentioned Fairview Health Services in Minnesota and Montefiore Medical Center in New York City, who have brought together the various stakeholders and participants in complex metropolitan settings to create greater capacity for integration and process rationalization. Montefiore is partnering with two other large hospital systems and two insurers in its community to work together on lowering hospital readmission rates by focusing on what happens to patients after they are discharged from the hospital.[11] Fairview Health Services has used a rapid innovation process involving many stakeholders to introduce innovations such as the development of twelve "care packages," which cover such medical concerns as prenatal care, kidney transplants, migraines, and hypertension. These are a way to provide consistent, high-quality care at a lower cost. All of Fairview's clinics are moving toward the "care packages" model (see sidebar).[12]

Much healthcare reform discussion focuses on accountable care organizations (ACOs) and medical homes as possible approaches to achieve system integration.[13] My hope for our profession is that we are actively involved in how this occurs, and in the many substantive integration tasks and innovative approaches. We all have to learn together, not just today and tomorrow, but into the future. Knowledge is proliferating and it is becoming possible to specify very high-quality pathways and guidelines. The field of healthcare is being impacted by many innovations that will lead to changes in how we are organized and how we do our work.[14] Those who learn and innovate will determine the shape of healthcare going forward.

Rapid Innovation and Redesign at Fairview Health Services

"Fairview used a rapid-iteration process to help our clinicians redesign the way health care is delivered, with an initial focus on primary care and creating a health care home for patients. What began as a pilot at two clinics has rolled out to forty primary care clinics. Physicians and staff are using team-based care and offering additional ways for patients to access care, including nurse-only visits, virtual care visits, and group appointments for some conditions.

We've added care coordination capabilities to manage care transitions across the entire continuum with a focus on patients with multiple chronic and complex conditions. We've invested in new technologies and data systems to manage care and patient transitions more effectively—including a unified medical record for our entire continuum. And, we've engaged specialists to develop 'care packages' to help standardize care and reduce costs for such conditions as low-back pain, diabetes, hypertension, and prenatal care. We are bending the cost curve."

—from "Changing the Way We Deliver and Pay for Care," by Mark A. Eustis.

Physician Lifetime Learning. Medical evidence is growing. New and more sophisticated diagnostic capabilities are proliferating. More targeted pharmaceuticals are being brought to the market. Surgeries have become more precise and less invasive. Physicians have a lot to keep up with! On the other hand, it is predicted that the better understood and more routine treatment of many conditions will be increasingly carried out with evidence-based, well-specified processes, and that many of the routine tasks now performed by physicians will be transferred to nurses, pharmacists and others. Physicians' roles increasingly will deal with more technically complex diagnostic decisions and clinical treatment.[15] Given the rapid advance of knowledge, the possibility of becoming obsolete is real. The only thing we know for sure about medicine in the future is that it will not be the same as it is today and that we need to keep up. We'll need innovative approaches to helping physicians keep up with the new knowledge and changes in healthcare.

Physicians have careers that last for decades. At SCPMG we take very seriously our obligation to our members, to the Kaiser Foundation Hospitals and Health Plan, and to each other to ensure that the physicians in our partnership remain educated in current methods and information. In addition to our core commitment to provide our physicians with ample educational time, we develop our own high-quality in–person and online courses that qualify for CME credit, and that prepare physicians for board recertification.

Our goal in these programs is to emphasize evidence and outcomes, and to make education as relevant as possible to physicians' practices. Given the busy schedules of doctors, we're introducing innovative approaches to doing this. The interactive webinar approach initiated by Dr. Marc Klau, the regional chief for Head and Neck Surgery, provides an efficient way for the head and neck surgeons in the region to learn about and discuss evidence, and to contribute to best practice guidelines. Physicians identify the topics, often because they recognize there is variation in practice and/or national guidelines are changing. A recent webinar focused on new national guidelines for pediatric tonsillectomy. Another will deal with the treatment of chronic sinusitis, a condition that costs six billion dollars in our country but where there is little agreement about the best care pathway. This webinar will involve both head and neck surgeons and primary care physicians. It will familiarize them with the evidence about best practices and increase their understanding about quality and outcomes issues in this area, as well as the financial costs of the current variation in practice. The discussion in the webinar will identify areas where the pathway needs to be better defined, and thus is highly relevant to key practice issues.

Although there are many virtual and in-person CME programs offered by national groups and vendors, we believe that our close linking of such programs to our physicians' practices and to our regional priorities accelerates changes in physician behavior and outcomes. Regional priorities are also evident in several of the other approaches we've developed. The "Pathway to Proficiency" course that we use to continually increase physician proficiency in the use of the EMR has physicians teaching other physicians how to use and get maximal benefit from the EMR system. Our region-wide commitment to educate our partnership about culturally responsive care addresses skills that we believe to be critical in today's multi-cultural world.

Our language concordance program (described in chapter three) is another innovation that addresses a key regional priority. It is aimed at matching patients with physicians who speak their language. It arose to address the quality risks that we faced because in about 26 percent of our visits, the physician and the patient couldn't speak directly to each other, but had to go through an interpreter. As part of the program we are committed to provide language training and even study-abroad opportunities for physicians who want to increase their language skills to qualify for the program.

Perhaps our most important educational innovation is SCPMG University. This program entails three day-long sessions during a physician's first six months with SCPMG. It is aimed at onboarding and teaching the philosophy of Permanente medicine. It focuses on our quality and outcomes objectives, practical information about possible pitfalls of practicing medicine and associated legal issues, and other topics of central importance to us, such as patient/clinician communication and the service ethic. During the courses, the physicians build a bond with other physicians from throughout the region, reinforcing the notion that we are one big team here to address the health needs of our membership. Since we have new physicians who come to us from medical schools all over the world and who have been trained in diverse settings, this program helps to create the common culture and expectation of career-long learning that is critical if any of our other innovations are going to succeed.

Empowering and Motivating Patients to Manage Their Health

The empowerment of patients to manage their own healthcare is another of the emerging trends that will help define a more sustainable healthcare system for the future. Innovations that facilitate this self-management have been one of our core focuses. The Internet has brought a previously unimaginable capability to tightly knit patient education and self-management into healthcare. I believe that we physicians must see it as part of our job to develop ways to actively incorporate this into our practices, rather than seeing it as something that is happening independently of us. We have developed a vast array of online and in-person courses, access to support groups, online diagnostics, and health information. These are not only aids to our patients who want to stay as healthy as possible, but also to our physicians who want to help them do so.

A patient can go online and take a survey about his back pain. From this self-diagnosis, he may identify an exercise plan to help with the pain or find out that his survey results indicate that he should visit a doctor. On the same kp.org website, he can schedule the appointment. Kp.org also has a wealth of information on healthy lifestyles. Additionally, patients can also be referred to health coaches via our Health Living Helpline to help them stop smoking, lose weight, or engage in an exercise regimen and manage stress. These coaches are members of our staff and are integrated into the patient's care team and their information flows into the patient's EMR. The most innovative aspect of these resources is the extent to which they are integrated into the patient's care plans.

Through access to their medical record and various applications such as scheduling and access to test results and care gaps, patients have new control over touch points with physicians and indeed with the whole healthcare system. We encourage all of our members to take a health risk assessment (HRA) and undergo biometric screening tests. This gives them an opportunity to better understand their risk factors and make the necessary changes to improve their health. Patients also have control over the modalities they use to communicate with physicians and other providers, and how they want to receive information.

We're also working with employers to introduce programs to help keep their most valued resource, their employees, healthy. We can create an aggregate report for a company on lifestyle and illness trends among their employees that helps them target initiatives to raise their employees' health level. And we can help them bring wellness programs and clinical care to the worksite. This allows the employees to choose whether to come to us for these services, or to receive them more conveniently at work.

Physicians are involved in crafting these various approaches to empower the patient. They're based on good medical evidence and also on evidence about communication and behavior change. Our researchers study these various approaches to see which lead to patient satisfaction, and which are associated with improved health outcomes. Thus, even these approaches are informed by evidence, and we're gathering the evidence to continually improve them. We see this as part of our Complete Care model.

Physician-Led Innovation

Reform of the healthcare system demands physician leadership and involvement in the development of new approaches. Physician leaders and front-line physicians at SCPMG have been integral to the crafting of the innovations described in this chapter. Our purpose has been to make changes that increase quality of care and value. A major tenet is to increase the effectiveness of the whole team, and thus the richness of the resources that enhance the impact of the work of the physician. We have been guided by the principle that we want to free up physicians to do physicians' work, and not weigh them down with tasks that can be carried out by a skilled healthcare team.

Healthcare needs continuing innovation to ensure that we are using the skills and resources of our healthcare system to best meet the needs of our patients, and to continually generate new knowledge and develop increasingly effective treatments. The four areas in which we at SCPMG have focused our innovation are designed to help us become a stronger system moving into an unknown future for healthcare and for physicians. Given the challenges we face, the changes we're introducing are sometimes disruptive to our comfortable patterns of practice. But, given physicians' critical roles in the healthcare system, our knowledge and perspectives are critical to successful innovation. All of us will not be innovators, but we need physicians who innovate and blaze the path for others. Implementing proven new approaches to increase value is the responsibility of all physicians.

Trend	Implications for Physicians	Am I effectively dealing with this trend now?
Value		
	1. We can only slow the increasing costs of healthcare through innovation. 2. Increasing quality of care and outcomes goes hand in hand with keeping people well. 3. Value can only be increased if doctors are involved in rethinking and championing new approaches to the way we work.	
Need for Innovation		
	1. Enhanced value demands: • proactive care • lifecycle approaches • continuous learning • empowering patients	
Empowered Patients		
	1. Patients want a variety of convenient ways to get health information: Online education, in-person courses, support groups are all important avenues for empowering them. 2. Patients want a variety of ways to access the system and communicate with their physicians and other caregivers.	

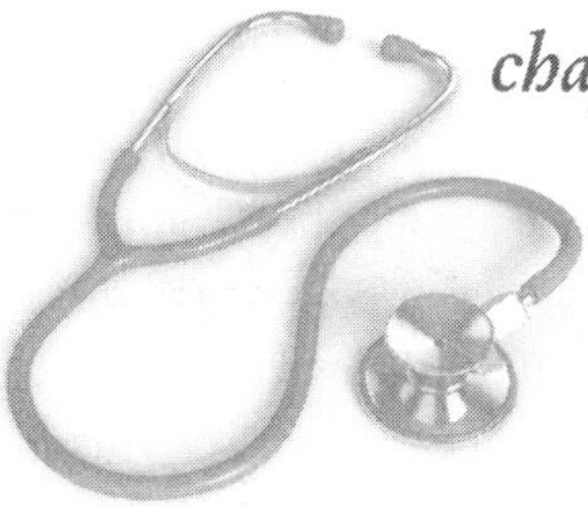

chapter eight

Integration and Teamwork

The societies in which we practice medicine have become much more complex, and we need to work differently to meet their needs. We need increased teamwork and integration of the many currently fragmented tasks and knowledge bases that are required to deliver care. Life is faster-paced, customers demand high performance, and they use their purchasing power to secure it. Industry after industry has had to go up the learning curve to deliver more value while consuming fewer resources. Now it's healthcare's turn. Traditionally designed, segmented approaches build in too much redundancy, coordination costs, quality problems, and they are far too slow to meet customer expectations. This has been frustrating for physicians, as well as for patients and their families. Yet I'm optimistic, because we are learning how to use the whole team more effectively.

Emerging models of healthcare require more reliable connections between providers in different disciplines and greatly increased teamwork to deliver integrated care. Teamwork is essential to build effective accountable care organizations and medical homes. When patients spend their time and money going lockstep through a linear sequence of uncoordinated care steps, they are not getting good care or good value. Perhaps even more importantly, such segmentation among providers locks in the inefficient status quo and keeps the healthcare system from learning and improving. As a result, society spends more and more on mediocre healthcare, as healthcare needs keep increasing.

Traditional organizations in all sectors of the economy were based upon functional and discipline-based departments, hierarchies, and individual responsibilities and accountabilities, and were built for stability and continuity, and for a simpler world. People only had to worry about their narrow job descriptions and not about working collaboratively with others. In the computer industry, the designer worried about the hardware design, but not about the cost of manufacturing it. The software developer made sure the software could operate without bugs, but didn't worry about ease of user interface. Customers were willing to pay for an expensive machine that didn't use resources efficiently, including their own time. But that didn't last for very long, because Apple learned how to design an efficient and powerful machine that was easy to use, and paid relentless attention to quality and the cost of manufacturing. It did this by working cross-functionally to optimize all the aspects of the design and manufacture of a machine that appealed to users. Meanwhile Dell Computer learned how to deliver a completely customized machine to customers within forty-eight hours. Suddenly many technical organizations—filled with bright, highly educated and often proudly independent scientists and engineers—had to organize so these highly skilled professionals would work together with a common vision and use resources wisely.

ACOs and medical homes are among the approaches that are being implemented to achieve the benefits of collaboration and coordinated care. In the 2010 healthcare reform law, the network of doctors and hospitals that form an ACO will be eligible for performance incentives if it agrees to manage all of the healthcare needs of a minimum of five thousand Medicare beneficiaries for at least three years and achieves targeted performance.[1] Premier and the Brookings-Dartmouth ACO collaborative are each leading collaboratives of healthcare organizations and sponsoring pilots aimed at learning how fragmented healthcare systems or healthcare eco-systems can reconfigure to meet the government requirements to be an ACO.[2] The concept of the medical home has been around for several decades and is aimed at providing coordinated, comprehensive medical care, often for youth, the chronically ill, or families.[3] The use of medical homes is increasing.

Granted, KPSC is a fully integrated system, but we have nonetheless historically suffered from the lack of coordination. In dealing with these issues, at KPSC we have been transitioning to team-based, complete care systems. Our teams can cut across organizational boundaries and include many disciplines, and are often virtual. They allow work to be coordinated in real time, and steps in the care process that used to be sequential can now be done in parallel. Teams are also used to define and implement change. As a result, changes can be made more rapidly, and the organization can innovate much more easily than a traditional organization.

In the business world, organizations have been using team approaches as a critical operating component for several decades, and they have been moving to increasingly networked and virtual ways of carrying out complex work. After many decades of resisting the use of teams, healthcare has discovered that it can't address the problems it faces without organizing differently to get more coordination and more innovation. We are just in the starting block of the marathon of change that other industries have already experienced.

These changes profoundly impact what it means to be a physician. Doctors are no longer lone wolves taking on the entire burden of care, hiring others to work for us, and seeing hospitals and other care delivery venues as resources in a physician-centric view of the delivery of care. This may have been an option at some point in history, but in today's continuously changing world, this stance is neither realistic nor effective. The fact is, physicians work as part of a network of care providers. If the teams we're in and the relationships we build are ineffective, so are we. It's no longer possible to say, "I'm a physician, and this is how I practice, and all others (including patients) should adapt to how I want to do business." To use our time and society's healthcare dollars wisely, we need to better coordinate to avoid quality problems and redundancy.

Doctors are no longer lone wolves taking on the entire burden of care, hiring others to work for us, and seeing hospitals and other care delivery venues as resources in a physician-centric view of the delivery of care.

As you have undoubtedly noticed in the preceding chapters, healthcare in the KPSC system has become a group effort. Our SCPMG physicians have led the way, finding ways to work with each other and across our system to improve the quality and value of care. Our system has evolved to include many kinds of teams. Teamwork helps push us all to greatness.

As healthcare processes become more coordinated, physicians everywhere can expect that they will be practicing medicine as members of teams. KPSC uses three kinds of teams that I believe are each important: 1) teams to make sure that the different institutional elements work together to optimize the whole system; 2) teams for the delivery of care; and 3) teams for innovation and improvement, including the rapid incorporation of evidence and best practice into the system.

Cross-Institutional Teaming: The Framework for Collaboration

Physicians increasingly are working in settings where institutional partnership is critical, but often missing. Those who fund healthcare, administer it, and operate hospitals, pharmacies, diagnostic and skilled nursing centers, and specialty clinics play critical roles in providing necessary services to patients. Physicians depend on all of these institutions in providing clinical care; indeed, clinical processes often cut across them. We *all* make decisions that affect one another, determine the patient's course of care, and impact outcomes. How well we work together determines whether good value is delivered for the healthcare dollar and good quality to the patient. Yet we are often separate departments and even different legal entities, each trying to push work onto the other's plate and maximize our own revenue flow.

Many healthcare systems are working to achieve greater integration between the various elements of care. Over the past years, the Cleveland Clinic has restructured into cross-functional organ- or disease-system institutes such as the Heart and Vascular Institute, OB-GYN and Women's Health Institute, and Pediatric and the Children's Hospital. Each institute provides patient-focused, integrated care, and has collective accountability for the value of care among the different specialties who get involved.[4] The Virginia Mason Medical Center in Seattle has evolved a process they call "marketplace collaboratives." They work with employers, health plans, and the providers from their multi-specialty system to define quality and build optimized clinical value streams in order to enhance quality, increase patient access, and reduce costs for providers and purchasers.[5] Systems such as Fairview in Minnesota and Montefiore in New York City are taking similarly collaborative approaches to integrate care delivery involving many participants who are not in an integrated system.

The Southern California Permanente Medical Group is a legally independent group, with an exclusive contract that is an annual agreement to deliver physician services to members of the Southern California Region of Kaiser Foundation Health Plan, in conjunction with the Kaiser Foundation Hospitals. Our long term relationship has contributed to our collective ability to optimize value by integrating care. We continue to look for ways to more fully take advantage of our collaborative potential.

I have been fortunate to work with a remarkable partner, Dr. Ben Chu, who leads the Kaiser Foundation Health Plan & Hospitals for the Southern California Region. We both knew that the only way to address the demands facing healthcare today was to fully align our region's resources to achieve prevention-oriented, integrated care. We knew we had the opportunity to fundamentally change the way we deliver medical care to enhance the capabilities of the whole system, and to create a win-win for all of us, but most especially for the members we serve. Our close working relationship has set the tone for teaming throughout the system.

As we all know, the finances of healthcare reform are paramount, and the various groups impacted by reform quickly fixate on who will get what resources. Yet our region did not begin our journey by mandating budget reductions or by making arbitrary decisions about who would get what. By working more collaboratively, we have found efficiencies that at the same time improve our quality, service, and outcomes.

Dr. Jeffrey Selevan, SCPMG's medical director for Business Management, has worked closely with the Health Plan on the evolution of the overall business model and even on the various elements of the health plan products. He started with the important premise that the physicians of SCPMG would and should only accept benefit designs that aligned financial incentives and were consistent with maintaining or improving quality of care. The strength of this long-term relationship depends on ensuring that all stakeholders align around a financial model that leads to ever-improving quality care while being excellent stewards of healthcare dollars. This required finding ways to achieve financial alignment between the region's Health Plan organization, the purchasers, the hospitals, and the medical group collectively. This alignment of incentives makes the quality, outcome, *and* efficiency goals of the system possible. Dr. Selevan did some very complex modeling of how all the factors come together, the impact of various changes on the overall capacity of the system, and how specific decisions relating to benefits or risk sharing result in favorable outcomes for the organization and for the members it serves.

The Ripple Effect of Institutional Collaboration

Dr. Todd Sachs, Chief of Surgery for West Los Angeles

"Jeff Weisz and Ben Chu came into their roles together eight years ago. They forged a relationship from the get-go and they were connected and a team. That has filtered down to everyone. We are not silos—the health plan and hospitals and SCPMG. We are taking the teamwork to the next level, whether at locations such as the OR, or in how we work together around a disease process. Redesigning the emergency room, putting a program in for bariatric control. You can't do it by yourself. You need all the intellectual frameworks. Recently I have been working more with the health plan. I love it. I wouldn't have been able to start the bariatric program without the support of people all the way to the Oakland board."

Dr. Brian Nguyen, Physician Director of Clinical Strategic Goals Optimization

"Part of our DNA is SCPMG coexists with the health plan. We all gain by how efficient we can make the system. We don't make more money by seeing more patients. But can we do what we're doing with cost savings while improving quality? That's important to our patients."

Physicians are very good at specifying what we need in order to deliver quality care. In order to build a sustainable model in today's world, we also had to step up to the plate and embrace the service and financial goals of the entire healthcare system, which in our case includes the hospitals and health plan organizations. Dr. Selevan's work helped us see how these parts fit together. The teaming relationship that has been established among the leaders of SCPMG and Kaiser Foundation Health Plan and Hospitals provides a foundation of shared goals and mutual trust of the decisions that are made about health plan products and benefits, capital and other strategic investments, and about the complex allocation of budget and shared risk for the region. The working relationship is based on the mutual purpose to provide quality care.

Shared goals and mutual trust also began to permeate the system as we worked together to make substantive changes in the way we approached healthcare for our members. According to Dr. Selevan, "We have learned to rely on a good relationship based on mutual trust and aligned goals so that we can work together to find solutions. Being able to identify and solve for mutually beneficial behavior between the entities is the magic that makes this work."

One of the earliest manifestations of the power of cross-institutional collaboration was the implementation of Kaiser Permanente's EMR system, HealthConnect. This was a mammoth national undertaking by KP, and one that was forward looking and even visionary in its scale and scope. As in other systems that have implemented an EMR, it involved extensive disruption to the way physicians had practiced and care was delivered, even while providing the tools to greatly increase quality. It certainly did stir up lots of strong feelings on the part of our physicians. Implementing the EMR required a system-wide effort just to get to the point where people could use the system effectively, and to tweak the system so it would operate to fit our needs. But it also provided us with evidence that we could all work together to effect significant and, at the time, quite overwhelming change.

In addition to the massive implementation plan that entailed extensive training and examination of the workflow, physicians who took quickly to the electronic system began teaching other physicians how to use it. Teams of physicians shared their ideas about how to make this system work effectively for them, and how to derive more benefit from it. We took their concerns seriously and spent a great deal of time and resources fixing things. And we went a lot further. We knew that the EMR would enable other changes that would make us better physicians and result in our system delivering enhanced healthcare. Many teams of physicians and other stakeholders became involved in making this happen quickly.

Cross-discipline teams across the region set to work to integrate many of our specialty legacy systems, such as our pharmacy system and our radiology system, with the core EMR. We drew on expertise throughout the system to reshape our registries to be compatible with the EMR, and to turn them into a powerful tool to improve care and develop the capacity to use our vast data to do comparative effectiveness research to advance clinical knowledge. Teams solicited and responded to hundreds of suggestions from physicians about changes and enhancements to our systems that would enhance their ability and the ability of their clinical teams to deliver great healthcare. There were no sacred cows. It would be naïve to think that installing such a huge edifice as an EMR in an organization would not affect practically everything else—nor that it could be accomplished without organization-wide collaboration.

Institutional teaming is also evident in our region's approach to quality and risk. Dr. Michael Kanter, SCPMG's medical director of Quality and Clinical Analysis and Patti Harvey, senior vice president for Quality and Risk Management for Southern California Kaiser Health Plans and Hospitals, work together closely, and collaboratively lead many initiatives throughout the region that have dramatically improved our quality of care. System-wide quality goals are aligned for SCPMG and the Health Plans and Hospitals organizations. Physician leaders in each of our thirteen area medical centers partner with their administrative team and nursing leaders to work through the trade-offs inherent in deciding how best to organize to deliver care. They jointly champion the teams that generate innovations and lead the implementation of change.

Institutional collaboration has resulted in our physicians being more willing to try new approaches and trust that the outcomes will benefit the whole system. Dr. Julia Bae, the medical director in Kern County, comments that this foundation of teaming between SCPMG and the Health Plan and Hospitals organizations has led to a greater flexibility in making service and quality related changes. Kern County is a rapidly growing area, and the physicians have been able to work with the Health Plan and Hospitals to make change fluid rather than adhering to strict negotiated budget constraints. "We have a long-term relationship with the Health Plan that allows us to trust that we'll all do our share," comments Dr. Bae. "Our medical group will cover an expense this time and we know that the Health Plan will invest in equipment we need in the future."

Teams for the Delivery of Care

Information is usually cited as a key to better and more effective teamwork.[6] With an EMR like ours, information is not in short supply. Networked information, such as is available via an EMR system, makes it possible for roles to be more flexible and the boundaries between our departments to be more permeable.[7] And in dealing with our patients, boundaries between our departments are definitely permeable. In Kaiser Permanente, our patients can show up anywhere in our system and get care. We have been developing approaches to create a complete integrated care system that enables us to operate as one big virtual team working in a coordinated manner. Our integrated IT systems underpin our Proactive Office Encounter systems that task people throughout the system with helping patients who come into our system to get their care gaps filled. The HealthConnect system facilitates our extensive targeted outreach to members, which provides them with important health information and reminders of screenings and tests they should undergo in order to be as healthy as possible.

Learning how to take advantage of HealthConnect to deliver better care is enabling us to revamp how we do work—and how we work together. It enabled us to use resources more effectively because we streamlined operations by giving a lot of responsibility to nurses, medical assistants, and back office staff to carry out tasks that were originally handled by the physician. We identified the transactional tasks that didn't need to be done by a physician, and systematically built them into the roles of nurses, pharmacists, medical assistants, receptionists, and many others groups in the system. All of our jobs have changed, to some extent, and I think for the better. Now, the whole team has information and is empowered and accountable for delivering patient-focused care.

Reinforcements for Primary Care. The predicted national shortage of forty-six thousand primary care physicians by the year 2025 is coming—just at the time when these physicians are increasingly central to emerging preventive and integrated models of healthcare.[8] Teaming primary care physicians with broadly trained support staff who can carry out many tasks required to deliver comprehensive primary care is an approach that is being used in many healthcare systems. Systems such as Medical Associates Clinics and Healthplans in Dubuque, Iowa, are creating "core teams" that partner physicians and nurses. The nurses carry out many of the tasks of preventive care and disease management, allowing the physicians to concentrate on diagnosis, disease treatment, and episodic care.[9]

As with healthcare nationwide, SCPMG faces the challenge of creating sustainable approaches to primary care. We were jolted as the medical literature began to report that a primary care physician with a panel of two thousand patients would require eighteen hours each day to take on the additional prevention tasks that we know are important for our members' well-being.[10] Working with a team of physicians, Nancy Spiegel, our head of Leadership and Organizational Development and Drs. Minardi and Kanter were able to identify literally hundreds of areas that were barriers to care, or where primary care physicians needed greater support or were doing work that did not require their expertise. Reminding patients that they are due for a screening exam or that they are due for their LDL (low density lipoprotein) test, for example, can be done by our highly trained support staff if they have the needed information from the EMR, and if the workflow is set up for this. Our team-based care system is similar to what is today more broadly called medical homes. A group of physicians, RNs, a pharmacist, MAs, and back office staff collectively take responsibility for the proactive management of care of their panels. The members of the team are given accountability for parts of the workflow—both in-reach and outreach–that fit their skills.

Some Teams at KPSC

- **Complete Care Teams:** Coordinate care of patients with chronic conditions
- **Proactive Office Encounter (POE) Teams:** Deliver team-based care
- **Unit-Based Teams (UBTs):** Natural work teams in hospitals and medical offices charged with levels of service quality and productivity, jointly sponsored by Kaiser Permanente and the Coalition of Kaiser Permanente Unions
- **Healthy Bones Care Team:** Assess bone density and manage care of those at risk for osteoporosis and fracture
- **Low Back Pain Care Team:** Multidisciplinary teams deal with episodes of acute low back pain
- **Arthritis:** Multidisciplinary team that defines care pathways, coordinated by orthopedic surgeons and care managers
- **Drug, Radiology and Lab Utilization Teams:** Regional multidisciplinary teams providing guidance to promote evidence-based use of critical resources
- **Proactive Inpatient Encounter (PIE)**
- **Case Management Team:** Deals with patients with complex conditions such as ESRD, HIV, and HF
- **Highly Reliable Surgical Teams**

Integrated Care Management Pathways. Teaming allows people with very different viewpoints, backgrounds, and expertise to bring their knowledge and skills to bear on the care of a patient. In working with a disease pathway or a complicated issue, this multiplicity of viewpoints can be a critical factor for success. Teaming allows us to look at a disease lifecycle or an acute illness more holistically through drawing upon each other's expertise.[11]

By working closely with the other groups in the system, including our pharmacy and analytical teams, Drs. Minardi and Kanter sponsored the development of care pathways that are connected to our registries, which are now closely linked to HealthConnect. Our care management systems link our various specialty groups in highly coordinated, proactive treatment of patients with chronic conditions such as diabetes, hypertension, asthma, or osteoporosis. Our Just-in-Time Clinics for the rapid assessment and intervention for those diagnosed with osteoporosis, and our team-based diagnosis and immediate treatment of patients with severe lower back pain are examples (described in chapter seven) where work once done sequentially through multiple visits is now being done in parallel by teams of providers.

Acute Care Process Definition. In our acute care systems, various physician leaders have been playing leadership roles in developing clearly defined team-based workflows. Through these initiatives, we have come to accept the importance of a standardized baseline to improving quality, safety, service, and productivity. We have been defining the flow and roles involved in preparing for, conducting, and delivering post-surgery care for both routine and complex surgeries. With leadership by Dr. James DeFontes, the assistant executive medical director in SCPMG Administration Perioperative Services, our Regional Perioperative Services have been redesigned around the concept of highly reliable surgical teams. These are cross functional teams, including surgeons, nurses, anesthesiologists, and all others involved in the full perioperative process starting with the initial contact with patient and family in the waiting room. The shared goal has been to align all the systems, people and processes to be the "safest place to have your surgery." For example, the members of our intact robotic surgery teams, including multiple physicians and highly skilled nurses and team leaders, have very precise roles and accountabilities that enable repeatable, highly reliable success. We know that all cases will have unique and somewhat uncertain elements, but we also know that the team can better deal with the unexpected if they are building on clear expectations of one another and of the core elements of the surgical process.

Unit-Based Teams (UBTs). In addition to the many process improvement activities being initiated by our SCPMG physicians, hundreds of improvement projects have also been initiated by Unit-Based Teams (UBTs). Unit-based teams are a primary workgroup at KPSC, consisting of all the participants in a natural work unit, including nurses, receptionists, doctors, supervisors, dieticians, phlebotomists, respiratory technicians, physical therapists, union representatives, and department administrators.[12] Examples of unit-based teams are a med-surge floor that might have twenty-four beds and fifty to eighty staff members, or a postpartum unit. Much of our workforce is unionized. KP's 2005 National Agreement with the Coalition of Kaiser Permanente Unions institutionalized unit-based teams and emphasized their role in making improvements to the way work is done.

> **Labor and Healthcare Improvement**
>
> John August, Executive Director of the Coalition of Kaiser Permanente Unions
>
> *"Unless you have the collective shared set of interests, nothing else is possible. There is a long history of employers in the healthcare industry trying to do quality improvement and until recently it has largely been a failure. A differentiator at Kaiser Permanente is that there has been an ownership of the strategy by the front line. Without that there will be top down initiatives that don't work. We worked hard on a shared sense of purpose."*

Rapid process improvement methodologies and a focus on lean functioning are integral to the improvement strategies of many premier healthcare systems. The Group Health Cooperative in Seattle uses them to target traditionally weak links in healthcare such as revamping how pharmacy delivers its services, and how patients are transitioned out of the hospital to other settings.[13] Intermountain Healthcare has used these methodologies for the improvement of more than one hundred clinical processes, and relies on teams consisting of physicians and nurses and others to lead the improvement processes. Nurses and physician leaders provide co-leadership in the clinical management structure that has been set up to ensure that these processes are implemented and ensure continual improvement.[14]

As part of the implementation of UBTs, our steering team visited many systems in the US and around the world to learn how to manage complex change. This included Jönköping County in Sweden, which had developed efficient ways to manage and govern more than fifty process improvements simultaneously. Through a highly participative process, it has become one of Europe's most effective healthcare delivery systems.[15]

KPSC has trained labor and management in systematic rapid process improvement methodologies. Our UBTs initiate improvement projects in pursuit of their service, quality, safety, and productivity goals. Many of our physicians become actively involved in these projects. The UBTs give the front-line workforce responsibility to come up with solutions and ideas to improve the patient experience, and to achieve regional goals. Patti Harvey, senior vice president for Quality and Risk Management for Southern California Kaiser Health Plans and Hospitals, notes that the front-line staff now better understand how they contribute from the patient and organizational perspective. "The organization is on a journey to empower the front line to take ownership over their processes." Physician leaders at each medical center are active in the UBT councils that sponsor the work.

According to Dr. Ed Ellison, who is my successor as executive medical director and chairman of the board of SCPMG, "By using various teaming approaches to improve processes, we are saying to our physicians, 'This is your practice. We need you to come together with the nursing staff and other support and talk about the issues you are facing. ' Often physicians are reluctant to have conversations with staff about what could be done differently to create a more effective practice. By using a systematic approach that includes the appropriate stakeholders, we can better define the work and create workplace agreements that improve our physicians' practices and benefit everyone."

Teams for Innovation: Building on the Evidence

We are at the front end of a fundamental transition in how healthcare is organized and delivered. As is apparent from the many examples throughout this book, there are literally hundreds of processes that must be reconceptualized for greater effectiveness. Most care pathways involve multiple specialty groups and units. For processes to be designed effectively and for changes to be accepted and implemented, the affected groups have to be involved in defining them. We need the right knowledge in the room. Yet we also have to learn from other units and other systems, and build on evidence in order not to overwhelm the system with redundant learning. Dissemination requires openness to learning from others' experiences and from their assessments of new approaches. We should stop trying to reinvent the wheel, and turn away from the "not invented here" syndrome. If evidence is to be incorporated into the way we carry out our work, physicians and others have to be involved in interpreting the evidence and translating it into practice. Many teams will be involved in defining, implementing, and disseminating the ongoing changes required to build a sustainable healthcare system.

I have given several examples where multidisciplinary teams have been used to improve our care processes, among them the Healthy Bones process, our diabetes and arthritis care pathways, and our lower back acute pain treatment process. Innovative processes are piloted and systematically assessed by innovation teams, first in one, and then in our other medical centers. Ultimately we build an evidence base that makes us comfortable that these approaches deliver better outcomes for our patients, and result in a better use of resources.

Our registries, the combined registries of our national KP system, and broader national and global registries have enabled teams of physicians to carry out important comparative effectiveness research in important clinical areas. One example of this is our work with hematuria, which began in 2007. Despite the frequent occurrence of hematuria in the population, there were no definitive evidence-based recommendations on how to proceed. To advance knowledge and treatment in this area, urology chiefs of service from all of the Permanente Medical Groups established a multidisciplinary team of physicians, including urology, primary care, laboratory, and radiology, to carry out a large retrospective study using the longitudinal KP database. They worked with the departments of guideline development, continuing medical education, and HealthConnect implementation to issue practice guidelines and publish the findings. (See sidebar, page 160.) These guidelines have avoided many unnecessary tests and much patient anxiety.

We also use teams of physicians to help incorporate new practices throughout the region. In 2005, our OB-GYN chiefs of service group identified the transition to greater use of minimally invasive surgery for hysterectomies as a key priority and an area where we could lead the nation. At the time, 38 percent of our hysterectomies were conducted in this way compared to a national average of 33 percent. A team of our gynecologists, who were experts in such surgeries, was brought together to develop a plan for region-wide proficiency. Working with our regional education and clinical consulting groups, they developed and taught a course for the other gynecologists throughout SCPMG on how to carry out minimally invasive laparoscopic and vaginal hysterectomies. It was a "mobile" course, offered in each of the region's thirteen medical centers. More than 80 percent of the region's hysterectomies are now minimally invasive, and we are leading the nation in this area.

Resource Utilization Teams

In chapter six, I talked about the importance of having approaches to continually and systematically introduce evidence into medical practices today. I gave the example of our Drug Utilization Action Team (DUAT). This

Hematuria

The Problem:

- Red blood cells in the urine are estimated to be the reason for 20% of all urology visits.[16]
- There have been no definitive evidence-based recommendations on how to deal with it.
- In 2007, there were conflicting recommendations from the AUA and from CUA.[17]
- This results in practice variation among doctors, and
- Many patients may be subjected to radiation and tests that they do not actually need.

The Research Initiative:

- In 2007, Kaiser Permanente chiefs of urology nationwide came together identified this as a high priority issue.
- The goal was to create evidence-based hematuria practice recommendations for urologists
- They sponsored a retrospective population-based cohort study
- A cross-region and multidisciplinary study team of physicians was set up to steer and run the study
- Starting with 772,002 patients who had undergone microscopic urinalysis during the study period
- They longitudinally tracked patients who had been found to have microhematuria, using the conventionally accepted level of 3 RBC/HPF.[18]

Findings:

After three years the overall incidence of urinary tract cancer differed from the general population rate only in men older than forty years with RBC/HPF greater than three and women over forty with greater than twenty-five (see Howard Jung et al.'s article "Association of Hematuria on Microscopic Urinalysis and Rick of Urinary Tract Cancer" for complete findings).

Products:

- A Standardized Hematuria Evaluation Practice Resource, which offers five recommendations, as well as resources and additional information, to practitioners when confronted with hematuria.
- Tools to help urologists work with the Resource
- CME materials
- HealthConnect diagnostic support[19]

physician-led multidisciplinary team is the region's nerve center for ensuring that we identify key issues in drug utilization, bring in the most up-to-date evidence about safety and efficacy, educate our physicians about the issues, and have region-wide metrics and vigilance about goals to support quality, safety, and cost effectiveness. DUAT is one of several teams that move us toward standardization by using evidence to inform our use of critical resources. What DUAT does with drugs, LUAT does with laboratory tests, and RUAT does with radiology. These are areas where new and expensive technology is continually being made available. Initially there are gaps in the evidence about which new approaches truly make a difference and about the associated safety issues. And there is a great variation of practice among physicians.

Like the DUAT, RUAT is a physician-led team that helps us to address a critical issue in medicine. In 2009, Americans had over 19,500 CT scans per day.[20] It was projected that twenty-nine thousand cancers would come into existence in the US as a result of the estimated seventy-two million CT scans that were conducted in 2007 alone.[21] Of the average total radiation a typical US resident receives, over half of it comes from medical radiation; in 1980 that figure was less than one quarter.[22] The growing use of imaging is also a significant contributor to escalating healthcare costs. For all of these reasons, I believe we have a responsibility to make certain that we use imaging judiciously. RUAT identifies approaches to make sure this happens. At SCPMG in the last three years, we have kept the increase in imaging studies to about 3 percent yearly, even with increasing numbers of patients in our care. Nationally, the use of MRIs, PET, and CT scans tripled in the decade after 1996.[23]

RUAT includes physicians from across KP's Southern California region; this includes radiologists, emergency room physicians, primary care physicians, and other specialties that are high prescribers of imaging. The team is responsible for identifying and providing evidence-based guidance, particularly about imaging exams that inherently raise patient safety issues because of the amount of radiation from the exam and/or because of the repetitive administration of radiation through time with questionable diagnostic or treatment advantage. Clearly these imaging procedures can give doctors a great deal of knowledge and visibility into a patient's condition, and they are an indispensable part of high-quality medicine. But they also entail a significant amount of radiation, and can put patients at risk. RUAT guidelines are not intended to constrain a physician's decisions with respect to a particular patient, but rather to provide a foundation to ensure overall appropriate usage patterns. RUAT metrics are part of our Vital Signs scorecard that goes to all our medical centers and departments (see chapter five on Goals, Measurement, and Accountability).

It Takes a Team

Our many team-based approaches are part of our complete care approach to deliver high-quality, integrated, and prevention-oriented care to our members, and to reduce the demands on the system for acute care and treatment of conditions that didn't need to get out of control and safety incidents that could have been prevented. Teams are integral to the continual improvement of outcomes and value. In today's world, doctors can't do all the tasks that are possible to enhance patients' health, and it is increasingly difficult to keep up to date with current practice. Doctors who try to go it alone are going to be very dissatisfied with work-life balance. We have to share the load and rely on our team.

Physicians today are overwhelmed by the demands on them in a world where in-baskets are full of messages from and about patients, where patients expect timely attention, and where every step is transparent and effectiveness is being measured and published. That's the reason that many of our physicians continue to become involved in improving our workflows, despite the fact that this means spending time participating in more teams, initiatives, and pilots. We have found that once we participate in defining effective workflows, our workload becomes more predictable and manageable. We see the results in terms of improved quality of life for our patients, enhanced quality and safety, and lives saved; this results in professional satisfaction for all of us. We have come to understand that dealing with the complexity of today's healthcare environment requires developing more effective and efficient ways to deliver care, and that this means a change in the way we work with other physicians and with the many other groups that depend on each other to deliver high-quality healthcare.

Trend	Implications for Physicians	Am I effectively dealing with this trend now?
Discontinuous and Increasing Velocity of Change		
	1. Delivering healthcare that meets society's needs and means demands greater coordination. The traditional segmented organization is slow, inefficient, and ineffective at delivering outcomes. 2. Working in multidisciplinary teams will become even more common. 3. Working collaboratively across organizational boundaries will become necessary for success (e.g., hospitals, insurance companies, IT, pharmacy).	
Teams for Improvement and Redesign of Healthcare Systems		
	1. Physicians are key participants in the teams that will find new ways to deliver care, and new ways to organize resources for greater impact.	
Coordination of Care		
	1. Effective use of healthcare resources requires more flexible roles and permeable boundaries. 2. Care pathways involve real-time coordination between many specialties and roles.	
Communities for Learning		
	1. Physicians learn from others' experiences and new approaches. 2. Teams help incorporate new practices.	

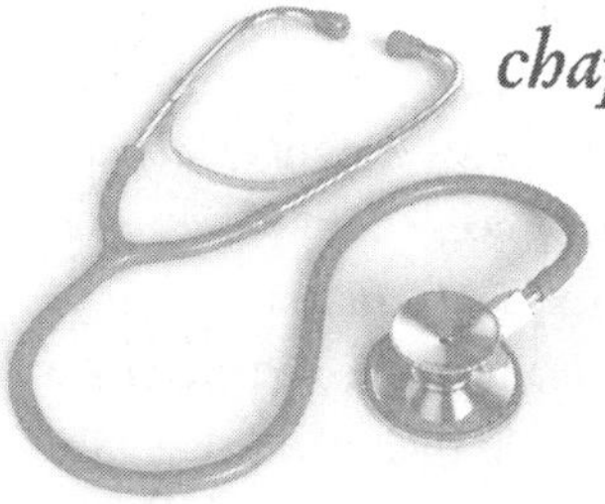

chapter nine

A Call to Action: Physicians Must Lead the Way

It's an exciting time to be a physician. New knowledge and medical technologies continually advance our capabilities to treat, cure, and prevent illness. Information technology enables new levels of integration of care and makes it increasingly possible to move many aspects of healthcare out of the rigid confines of doctors' offices and to venues and modalities that better fit the patient's life. Patients are increasingly well educated about health issues and able to partner with us in their care.

Yet societal and economic pressures on our healthcare system grow faster than our resources, and our traditional approaches to delivering healthcare are under attack. I believe we can create healthcare systems that truly deliver high-value healthcare. Leading such change is an opportunity. It's also an imperative.

Sustainable healthcare systems can be built only if physicians lead the transformation, and if we are leaders in the teams and systems that deliver healthcare. This is really a change in our identity. We were trained to deliver healthcare, not to lead. Our peers respect us for our clinical capabilities, not our leadership acumen. We expect that society will accept our judgment and do our bidding because of our expertise and skills, and that healthcare delivery systems will be organized around us. After all, we're the most important actors in the system. Aren't we? We have come to expect that all the support we need will be provided, and we complain when that doesn't happen.

Funding? That's "their" problem. Some may enter the healthcare reform fray mostly to protect physician interests—including autonomy and income. And when those who pay for our services say "no," we may cry foul and protest that practicing medicine isn't what it used to be. Perhaps we feel singled out and picked on, as if any other occupation is what it used to be!

> **Making the Physician's Voice Heard**
>
> Dr. Todd Sachs, Chief of Surgery for West Los Angeles
>
> *"As we progress into the future, we need to ensure that government actions related to health care reflect the physician's voice. Physicians should step up and realize they play an important role in decision making for the betterment of patient care."*

Not a pretty picture, to be sure. Yet I'm optimistic because I have seen what can happen when physicians accept that we are part of a complex healthcare system, and when we become leaders for change. I believe that new physicians starting out in their practice gladly embrace a system that is built to take advantage of new capabilities and to have greater impact. And I've found throughout the system I've been leading that many physicians are energized by the chance to build a system that truly works to deliver affordable, high-quality healthcare to our patients: a system designed for health.

If you're entering the field of healthcare right now, the chances are almost 100 percent that you'll become part of a system in transition. You'll be part of defining the future. The system you help build may look and operate quite differently than the integrated system that I have been part of and have described in this book. But it will be different than the status quo. It has to be. The status quo is not accomplishing the outcomes our society needs and demands. Are you proud to be part of a national healthcare system that costs twice as much per capita as other countries, yet yields mediocre results? I'm not.

Being part of an effective system is gratifying for everyone. In specialty area after specialty area, I've seen the pride that ensues when physicians set out to move the needle on outcomes, and when performance rises dramatically. SCPMG's thirteen chiefs of obstetrics and gynecology, for example, have systematically built a region-wide strategy for addressing the high-priority areas impacting women's health. Our gynecological practice has become a national leader in areas such as minimally invasive surgery and is developing region-wide centers of excellence for reproductive endocrinology and infertility. They've modeled demand and supply of resources and are developing systematic care delivery models. Dr. Teresa Wray, the regional chief of OB-GYN, reports the increase in pride that the physicians feel in the measurable accomplishments and "in being part of a premier system." In specialty after specialty I've seen the collective pride that comes from identifying the highest priority focuses that can make us such a premier healthcare system, and from leading the many to get there.

In the many healthcare organizations making great strides to create high-value healthcare, physicians have been integral to the change effort.[1] Physicians are assuming leadership roles in increasingly team-based healthcare delivery systems. These include the Cleveland Clinic, a premier research center and globally recognized fee-for-service healthcare system. Under the leadership of Dr. Delos (Toby) Cosgrove, it has transitioned from traditional medical and surgical divisions to multidisciplinary institutes to treat specific organ or disease systems. Its twenty-six physician-led institutes are charged with continual improvement of care that is collaboratively delivered and patient-centered. They are responsible for progress against clinical and cost objectives within the goals and strategies of the Clinic. The Clinic continues to be cited as one of the top ten systems in the country in most of its specialty areas.[2] Similarly, a public-sector health system, the Veterans' Health Administration, was reorganized into twenty-one networks, each with accountable physician leadership. This transition, led by Dr. Ken Kizer, has resulted in the VA becoming a leader in clinical quality, with a significantly lower risk of death for men over sixty-five and patient satisfaction 12 percent above the US average.[3]

Even in the day-to-day delivery of care, it's no longer sufficient for physicians to be highly skilled experts with a staff working for us. To deliver high-quality, patient-centered care, we have to be leaders in the diverse teams that serve our patients. To make preventive care a reality, we have to look more broadly at our patients and coordinate with other specialties and providers. To continually introduce evidence-based practice, we have to be part of strong multidisciplinary communities of practice. Strong communities of practice require strong leaders. To continually innovate and improve so we deliver increasing value, we have to be leaders in innovation and participate in the improvement of processes that are focused on the needs of the patient, quality, and efficiency. We can no longer ask that processes be fashioned around the way we want to practice medicine. And we can't afford to leave the improvements to others. We have to lead the way.

Senior Leadership

Throughout the book I've been describing physician-led projects that are transforming the nature of our healthcare system at KPSC. These have been occurring within an umbrella framework crafted by our senior leadership team, which is composed of extremely talented physician leaders who collectively envisioned new ways to use our resources to deliver greater value, and then worked collaboratively to put them in place.[4] We knew that we couldn't achieve a prevention orientation simply by heaping more and more tasks on our physicians. In order to deliver increased value, we had to distribute tasks differently to free up physicians from work that other team members could do just as effectively. Based on this principle, we developed our proactive approaches to deliver patient-centric, integrated care to different patient segments. Many physician leaders helped craft and implement these approaches.

Strategic leadership from the senior team has been critical in providing a vision and a path through the healthcare value challenges being faced by our society. The senior leaders have modeled a way of approaching the myriad of areas where change is needed. They quickly started to move the physicians in our partnership beyond the win-lose notions that had prevailed—and beyond their beliefs that increasing quality requires increasing resources. Members of the senior team provided a way of thinking about optimizing quality, service, cost, and outcomes *simultaneously*, and provided a model for the rest of the leaders in our system by aggressively pursuing this joint optimization. By combining the principles of rigorous measurement, evidence-based approaches, and financial modeling, they set the expectation that we could continually detect areas where we could increase quality while becoming more operationally efficient and eliminating non-value-added tasks. We could thus redirect scarce resources to improve medical care in the areas of prevention, quality, and service.

The principle is simple. *If we focus on what really makes a difference, we can increase the value delivered for the healthcare dollar.* Acting on this principle in the face of thousands of physicians with varying ideas about what makes a difference requires leaders who are dedicated to making it happen, and willing to be guided by evidence. Leaders have found ways to measure impact in terms of the outcomes most important to physicians and patients: lives saved, disease progression slowed, unnecessary hospitalizations and surgeries avoided, and quality of life enhanced. Throughout SCPMG, change momentum has been accomplished by creating common goals that have aligned the partners with each other and with the whole system. Without an aligned and respected physician leadership team, this would not have been possible.

Shared Leadership

Shared leadership is an essential principle in healthcare. Physicians, especially those in a partnership, do not respond to a command and control leadership style. In fact, when practicing physicians are appointed physician leaders, their partners may suddenly view them with a jaundiced eye because of their new title and role. This may be true even though they have worked side by side with their colleagues for years in a collegial fashion and have been respected for their clinical acumen and excellent medical care. Many physicians do not like to be led and resent others in their ranks who are promoted to leadership positions. They've "joined the other side" and are no longer "one of us." This makes it even more critical that there are physician leaders throughout the system who practice medicine and take the lead in making sure that we deliver the best possible care. Our physician leaders at SCPMG deeply understand and care passionately about having the freedom to do the best thing for our patients. We all appreciate and respect the meaning of "partner."

Changing physician behavior requires clinical leaders throughout the system who lead change that is based on evidence. At the end of the day, physicians will not adopt change unless it will result in better care. In our physician partnership, direction comes from peer consensus. A key task for a physician leader is building that consensus—around directions that can empirically be shown to be beneficial. And that's much easier to do if you continue to practice medicine and lead by example. That's why I think it is important for physician leaders to continue to practice medicine in order to help avoid the gulf between physicians in leadership roles and other physicians. You have to be seen as the one who rolls up his sleeves first and also are respected for your excellence and hard work as a physician.

Evidence underpins all true healthcare reform, and it also underpins physician leadership. Without evidence we cannot improve quality, outcomes, and value. Without evidence, we cannot and should not persuade physicians to change their practice. Physicians line up behind evidence, not exhortations. At SCPMG we have the attitude that if the evidence doesn't exist, we need to investigate and find it. Many leaders throughout SCPMG have become involved in initiating ideas, gathering the evidence, testing various approaches and generating new evidence, sharing learning, and determining practice guidelines and delivery models. This can't be done from leaders at the top. It requires clinical leaders throughout the system.

Leadership for Clinical Excellence

There are many formal and informal physician leadership opportunities in most healthcare systems. The quality of that leadership determines how well the system will succeed at moving from being a good solid system to a great one. This challenge has energized many of our chiefs, who have seized the opportunity to make a difference and have worked with their teams to identify opportunities to dramatically improve. Our regional chiefs of service have built region-wide and even national communities of practice. These chiefs are highly knowledgeable about the evidence in their fields, and are viewed as clinical practice leaders as well. They are also attuned to the importance of using resources wisely and delivering greater value. They champion the introduction of new evidence-based practices and the exploration of comparative effectiveness. They work with their colleagues in their specialty to define new standards of practice, disseminate best practice, and to innovate. They sponsor physician-led teams to explore and test new approaches.

We believe that a culture is being built that promotes the focus on excellence. Physicians throughout the region are identifying opportunities to improve processes, and to investigate and introduce new technologies. Dr. Jim DeFontes, our assistant executive medical director, SCPMG Administration Perioperative Services, believes that through our early successes, we are "building leaders who now want to continue to have this ongoing process improvement. We're asking, 'Where is the variation in outcomes as well as variation in practice?' And let's determine what is the best practice and put it in place. This way of working is driving itself without pressure from the top."

All physicians won't be innovators or lead process improvement teams, but new integrated approaches to medicine require most physicians to be daily leaders in front-line teams. Let's not forget, as soon as we put on the white coat, we are looked to for leadership.

The Desire to Innovate Is Infectious

Dr. Tad Funahashi came to Kaiser Permanente in Orange County to work with his mentor, Dr. Dale Daniel, who saw the tremendous potential for population-based research. He quickly realized that it was a great place to innovate.

"The previous medical director of Orange County, Dr. Ed Ellison, who is now the executive medical director of SCPMG, encouraged innovation and combined it with a focus on performance. His mantra was 'performance buys autonomy.'

Orange County collected a bunch of physicians of like mind. Once you get that milieu, innovation starts to happen. We make advances and begin to replicate them elsewhere. Excitement builds.

The Orange County senior leadership was trusting and provided the opportunity to do pilots. This feeds on itself and we identify many ways to get even better."

— Dr. Tad Funahashi, Regional Chief of Orthopedic Surgery, SCPMG.

Not only do we lead the care of the patients in our panels, but the healthcare team around us looks to us to set the example and direction for day-to-day care. Front-line teams include the teams that manage the care of a panel of patients, high-performance surgery teams, and care management teams for patients with chronic illness. Our front-line physicians also take part in the process improvements initiated by our unit-based teams throughout the system. The desire to innovate to have greater impact on our patients' health is infectious. We've found that as more and more physicians identify areas where we can deliver greater value to our patients—better outcomes, higher safety, more convenience, a better experience—more and more physician leaders emerge.

Leading Disruptive Change: Today's Challenge for Physician Leaders

Our physicians have had to deal with significant change in the past decade, much of which has been disruptive to their practice patterns. The introduction of the EMR, increased transparency of outcomes, and the changes in the service, quality, and value expectations of our many stakeholders have naturally made many physicians uneasy. We have experienced initial resistance to many of the changes we have implemented. The challenge faced by our SCPMG leadership team has been nonetheless to unlock the energies of our six thousand-plus physician group, and to continue to raise the bar for performance throughout our partnership.

Rewarding for Performance. When we expanded pay for performance eight years ago, there was a great deal of pushback by some of our physicians. The outcry consisted of, "We've never done it this way before, why now? You're going to ruin the foundation and culture of our medical group." Many physicians were comfortable with the philosophy that all of them should be paid equally within their discipline, regardless of the outcomes and care provided to their patients. Others feared that pay for quality performance was really a way to incent them to reduce costs, and that quality might suffer. Over a three to five year period, with a lot of hard work and a not insignificant amount of tension in the partnership, we have been able to overcome the resistance. Our physicians came to accept that the incentives are linked to issues that are central to our capability to deliver high-quality care to our members. It is now well accepted and part of our care delivery system—

not only for physicians but also for other providers in the system. As many physicians say, the amount of pay in the incentive is not very large, but the fact that it's there makes many of us sit up and take notice and more fully understand SCPMG's goals for delivering outstanding care. Now we're all striving toward the same goals.

KPSC's Values

- *Quality*
- *Service*
- *Results*
- *Integrity*
- *Partnership*
- *Diversity*
- *Accountability*
- *Flexibility*
- *Innovation*

Aligning Focus Through Performance Management. In my view, this change in the reward system was necessary to align physicians with the new realities of healthcare—and well worth fighting for. But to do this, we had to institute a performance management system that was designed by physicians, was viewed as fair, and that aligned the objectives of everyone in the system around the values that we stand for.

Feedback underpins the capacity to change and improve. The introduction of a strong performance management system based on metrics and priorities that have been defined by the partnership itself has been critical. We have built on KPSC's values. When I started here, we were strong in the areas of partnership, integrity, diversity, and quality, but needed to improve in results, service, flexibility, innovation and accountability. As we have stressed goals and metrics, transparent feedback, and a greater drive for performance and results (see chapter five), these lagging values were improved. Focusing on all of our nine values is leading us to affordable, high-quality healthcare where patients experience exceptional access and service.

In spite of clear evidence of large gains in quality, brand reputation, innovation, and a simultaneous increase in financial rewards for our physicians, these systematic approaches to managing performance were not always popular. In fact, there was a time in 2008 when it looked as if I would fail to win reelection as executive medical director of SCPMG. Leaders, particularly when pushing for higher standards and when moving people out of their comfort zone, have to have the stomach to take unpopular stands. By relentlessly emphasizing performance excellence, a leader can simultaneously confront the pushback and build on the partners' natural energies for excellence. Our performance management system has provided our physician leaders with the tools they need to address performance problems, and to reward outstanding performance. Physicians don't like to be perceived as low performers. Good comparative data, particularly about outcomes and resource consumption, provide the basis for feedback and discussion that can start to change behavior.

Confronting Pushback with Positive Forces. The aggressive implementation of our EMR was definitely a disruptive change for our physicians. Its implementation brought out many hostilities and caused great upheaval among our physicians. HealthConnect was an enormous system change. Dr. Ed Ellison, who is my successor as executive medical director of SCPMG, described the change leadership challenges he experienced as the medical director in the Orange County area, and how he dealt with them. He described his role as helping the physicians "getting past the valley of despair" (see sidebar).

Leaders of change have to pick the battles to wage, and look for the opportunities to pull out the positive forces. For the EMR, the positive forces included using younger, more tech-savvy physicians to help the others, and giving physicians the opportunity to help shape the development of the system. Pushing on with aggressive EMR implementation required strong leadership and yielded great benefits. The EMR has unleashed a torrent of ideas for how we could improve healthcare now that we have good data. We all have access to the same information, we can demonstrate impact, and we can continually improve based on sound assessments.

Data are critical to physician decision making. Aggressive implementation of the EMR

Getting Past the "Valley of Despair"—Introducing the EMR to Thousands of Physicians

"The organization did a good job in terms of training physicians. When we went live, there was a swarm of technicians surrounding our physicians to help. These technicians understood the product but not the care delivery process.

Fortunately, in Orange County we had a cadre of young, really tech-savvy physicians who took to the EMR quickly and who became our early adopters. Many of them had experienced an EMR in their training, and their expectation was that we have that same level of technology in place.

Many of my generation struggled with implementation, and for most physicians it took at least a year to become comfortable with the product. The improvements were slow during the first three to four months, creating what felt like 'a valley of despair.' Then we reached a milestone level where we could see that things actually did get better.

As a leader, I had to keep the hope alive. I encouraged learning from the areas that had progressed more quickly or where it had been introduced earlier. 'Your office is still in the start-up phase, but if you look at office X, three months ago they were where you are now and today they're running really smoothly. Go see what they did.' All the chiefs were extremely focused on EMR implementation for that year.

There was constant communication. We had off-sites so the physicians could suggest changes and learn from each other. We identified physician champions to help others. Our different physician groups brought in the early adopters to talk about what they did to get past the startup pain and use the EMR effectively.

Now for the most part, we wouldn't go back—we see the benefits. But it was a rough first year for our physicians."

— Dr. Ed Ellison, Executive Medical Director and Chairman of the Board, SCPMG

was the right battle to wage. It has provided our physicians with the opportunity to use data to identify important problems and opportunities, and to lead change. Without the systematic assessment of changes, it would be difficult to get our physicians to implement them.

The change to the EMR took us out of our comfort zone, and many (or most) of our physicians at the time were questioning the wisdom of taxing the system to the extent that was required for successful implementation. We even lost some physicians because of this. There was not yet a federal mandate to put such systems in place. We were ahead of most other systems, and there were few role models to suggest we could come out of this transition with greater capacity than we started. It just seemed like extra work. Strong leadership was required in all of our medical centers to offset the natural tendency to demand a return to the status quo. Without persevering through what Dr. Ellison called the "valley of despair"—while ever listening and responding to physician concerns and making changes to the system as appropriate—our system could not have derived the benefits that have allowed us to find many ways, large and small, to become more effective.

Trust and Openness. Many physicians are socialized to see other healthcare participants as the enemy. This often includes administrators, insurance companies, labor unions, and sometimes even nurses. Yet the truth is that the healthcare systems we depend on would grind to a halt without these groups. Without them, we would return to the day when the care a patient received was limited to what a single physician could provide in a private office, or to the era of public hospitals that were no more than holding pens for very sick people. We depend fundamentally on the work of the many specialty groups throughout the system. Yet we often don't trust the motives or competency of these other groups. Distrust has severely limited our ability to lead in the creation of the emerging healthcare system.

Strong leaders in all stakeholder groups are needed to establish the requisite levels of trust, collaboration, and coordination to deliver value. Our physicians have not always been comfortable with our close working relationship with the Hospitals and Health Plan organizations. Some feared that we might abandon physicians' interests. I didn't buy that. I saw no way that we could address the challenges facing us without building a strong relationship. I pursued that vigorously. By persevering and developing trust, collaboration is now extended into the entire region. We see strong partnerships blooming in local departments throughout the region between physician, nursing, and administrative leaders.

Trust is developing and enabling new ways of doing things that weren't possible in a time when our physicians did not believe that our administrative and labor counterparts would step up to the plate. Debbie Ogawa, a KPSC management consultant who has been working with teams designing high-performance surgical processes, notes the change, "The education for the physicians has been that when you set up a team where everyone has an equal voice, ideas come from peers and staff alike, and this leads to everyone accepting the innovations or changes, and doing their part. Physicians get caught up in the energy of the group. It really gets them on board when there is a systematic 'test of change' and they see how it made a difference." Slowly this trust is spreading through the region, as leaders model collaboration and sponsor, champion, and participate in joint initiatives and the development of highly integrated processes.

Developing Leaders

Leadership skills are not part of most physicians' training, yet in our system new physicians are almost immediately asked to assume leadership roles, particularly in their local teams. New physicians also may bring the most current knowledge of new techniques, and may be asked to help introduce them to the broader practice. If you're a relatively new physician, you may be learning how to practice and simultaneously learning how to lead a team or an initiative.

The need for physician leadership is being felt throughout the healthcare world. For example, HealthCare Partners, also based in Southern California, is a multispecialty medical group that sees developing its physicians as essential to the success of the organization. Dr. Robert Margolis, MD, the managing partner and CEO, says that, "Our future depends to a great extent on thoughtful physician leaders." To develop that leadership capability, the organization has had over a dozen of their physician leaders go through the California HealthCare Foundation Healthcare Leadership Program, which is a part-time, two-year development program. In addition, about two years ago, HealthCare Partners developed its own nine-month-long leadership development program, with between thirty and forty physician and managerial leaders taking part each year. The program teaches leadership skills and team skills, while also furthering the professional development of HealthCare Partners' core physician and management executives in its California,

Florida and Nevada divisions. Intermountain Healthcare's Institute for Health Care Delivery Research offers courses for practicing clinicians, senior leaders, and quality improvement leaders, including a twenty-day Advanced Training Program and a nine-day mini Advanced Training Program. The courses aim to develop participants' skills to lead, implement, and investigate quality improvement.[5]

At SCPMG, we benefit by being part of an organization that places value on the educational development of physician leaders through many internal and external programs. I personally benefited from attending the Stanford Program (a mini-MBA program), where I first came across Tushman and O'Reilly's *Winning Through Innovation* book.[6] I also attended the Chapel Hill, North Carolina advanced leadership program. We start providing development experiences at the early stages of a physician's career. Our new physicians attend SCPMG University and learn how to manage their practice, how to be leaders in their module teams, and how to work within an integrated healthcare system. SCPMG University emphasizes key characteristics of being a successful physician and caring for patients, and it sets high expectations on the necessary elements that are required to be a partner in our medical group. It lets our new doctors know the many ways a doctor can be a leader. They could be a quality leader, a board member, chair their medical center credentialing committee, or they could head up the drug utilization or hospital utilization group in their medical center. Opportunities abound. We encourage them all to mix leadership work with patient care. For physicians who have assumed formal clinical leadership roles (our chiefs), we offer a menu of courses on such topics as facilitated leadership, negotiation of conflict, and public speaking.

Physicians who are choosing where to practice medicine should investigate the resources that are available to help them become physician leaders. Given the amount of change coming down the pike, it would certainly be better to help shape it than to be buffeted around by it. In today's world, being a professional means so much more than having good technical skills, and leadership skills are certainly a major element.

In Conclusion

Our national healthcare system is unhealthy. We have some outstanding systems that deliver the best care in the world, yet we have a broad expanse of population who are not touched by effective, patient-focused, prevention-oriented care. We have a system oriented toward heroic treatment and not toward keeping people well. And we are spending too much money compared to the value derived by our citizens in general. Our patients suffer because physicians do not coordinate well with each other, carry out redundant tasks, and do not always keep up with the evidence. In addition, we often don't think about the whole person and what values each person holds dear.

And yet, I am optimistic. I believe we are coming to understand how healthcare can truly be reformed. We have to change the organization of healthcare and the roles of its many contributing stakeholders to take advantage of the astounding new clinical and technological capabilities that are now available. We can address our resource constraints if we begin to think increasingly about how to keep people well. We can deliver much more value if we begin to work together. We can achieve a healthier population while also reaping the economic benefits of delivering better care at lower cost.

Based on my experience leading SCPMG and working collaboratively with Kaiser Foundation Health Plan and Hospitals, I am optimistic that physicians are rising to the challenge, and will lead the way in the continual improvement of the capabilities of our healthcare systems. We all want to deliver on the promise of medicine and achieve better outcomes and a healthier population. KPSC has demonstrated this by delivering on our vision, the KP Promise, with its four cornerstones: quality you can trust, caring with a personal touch, convenient and easy access, and affordability.

Physicians working in poorly functioning healthcare systems cannot fully deliver on the promise of the astounding capabilities that are theoretically available to us. We can individually do wonderful and impressive feats in treating sick patients, but if the system beyond the confines of our office doors and our treatment rooms is not designed to support the full health of the patient, our impact is diminished. This system is not other people's responsibility; it is the responsibility of all of us.

In this book, I have developed my sense of the trends in healthcare that are shaping the system of the future. These trends provide the context to make significant leaps forward in how we deliver healthcare. We may not get there easily as a nation or even as individual healthcare systems. But ultimately we need to get there if we are to have a healthcare system that is a positive contributor to the quality of life of our citizens and the well-being of our societies and our economies. A healthy healthcare system also creates meaningful and satisfying work for healthcare providers. This is why I think it's a great time to be a physician.

I believe we will get there much more quickly and will arrive at a better destination if physicians are major players in shaping this system. My aim with this book has been to provide a realistic set of expectations about practicing medicine in today's world and to detail the trends and changes that physicians will have to deal with. I have also challenged our profession to become leaders in defining the new healthcare. We have a tremendous opportunity to make a difference. As I have argued throughout this book, I believe that the practice of medicine will be infinitely more gratifying if we are part of, and help create, high-performing systems focused on keeping people as healthy as possible.

For doctors already practicing, and for new physicians just coming into clinical practice, I wish you all the best. I hope that you will always remember why we're here: for the patient. Strive for excellence in your practice, never stop learning, and be a good leader. Take intelligent risks, and develop relationships with your colleagues and patients. Above all, speak and act from the heart.

Trend	Implications for Physicians	Am I effectively dealing with this trend now?
Opportunity to Lead the Way During a Time of Great Change		
	1. Medicine and society need physicians to take the lead in building a sustainable healthcare system. 2. Leadership of the care delivery team is an increasingly important physician role in integrated care pathways. 3. Physicians will increasingly lead system improvement initiatives—often working with the other parties in the healthcare space. 4. Physicians will have increasing opportunities to contribute to clinical learning and best practice development. 5. Senior physician leadership will increasingly use goals, pay for performance, and formal performance management systems to align physicians to achieve higher performance outcomes. 6. Leadership development opportunities are increasingly important for physician careers.	

Appendix 1

Southern California Progress in the Areas of the KP Promise

The vision of KPSC is the KP Promise. The KP Promise has guided our priorities and our metrics. It consists of these four elements:

- Quality you can trust
- Caring with a personal touch
- Convenient and easy access
- Affordability

Below are some key metrics and accomplishments that show our progress in the areas we track to ensure that we are making the KP Promise a reality.

Quality

Medicare HEDIS Rankings 2010 – Effectiveness of Care
KP Ranked in the Top 10 Nationally

- Controlling High Blood Pressure (#1)
- Osteoporosis Management in Women Who Had a Fracture (#1)
- Adult BMI Assessment
- Breast Cancer Screening
- Colorectal Cancer Screening
- Cholesterol Management CAD
  - LDL Screening
  - LDL Level < 100
- Comprehensive Diabetes Care
  - HbA1c Testing
  - LDL Screening
  - LDL Level < 100
  - Eye Exam
  - Medical Attention for Nephropathy (#1)
  - Blood Pressure Control
- Antidepressant Medication Management
  - Acute and Continuation Phase

HEDIS Data, compiled by SCPMG and Stakeholder Communications. (2011, October). "Accolades, Awards, and Accomplishments."

Figure 1: *Quality. Medicare HEDIS Rankings 2010 – Effectiveness of Care*

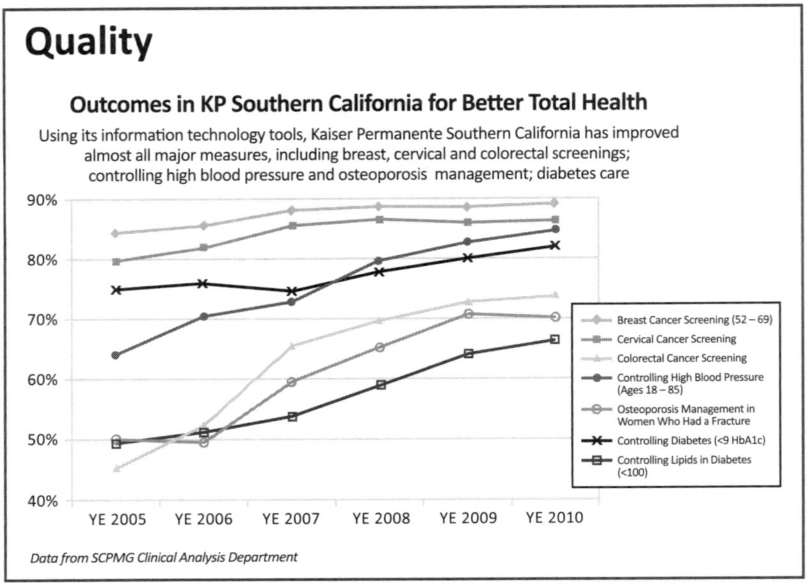

***Figure 2:** Quality. Outcomes in KP Southern California for Better Total Health*

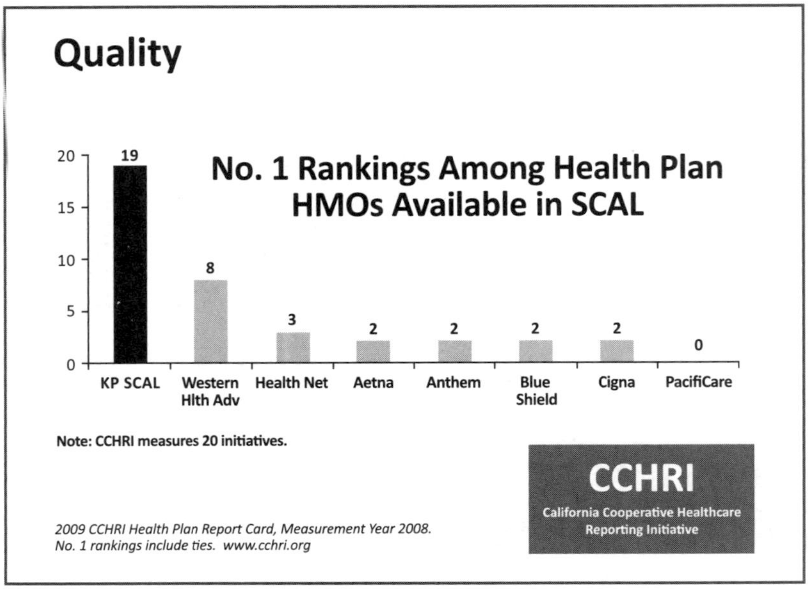

***Figure 3:** Quality. No. 1 Rankings Among Health Plan HMOs in SCAL*

Patient Care Experience

SO. CALIFORNIA: Members Rating KP	BASELINE 2004 SCORE	SPRING 2011 SCORE	INDEX SCORE* Spring 2011 / Baseline X 100
INDIVIDUAL BRAND ATTRIBUTES			
Excellent Care	80%	87%	110 ↑
Eady to Get What Need	73%	81% *All Time High*	111 ↑
Top-Notch MDs	74%	81%	109 ↑
Compassion	69%	83% *All Time High*	120 ↑
Affordable	75%	73%	97
Proactive	80%	85%	107 ↑
Innovator	65%	72%	111 ↑
Wide Choice	62%	71%	114 ↑
Health of Community	67%	79%	117 ↑
Leader in Online Access	88%	88%	100
GLOBAL BRAND ATTRIBUTES			
Overall Opinion	81%	88%	108 ↑
Changing for the Better	48%	55%	114 ↑
Intent to Renew	92%	95%	103
Recommend KP	52%	59%	115 ↑

↑↓ indicates significant change from Baseline to Current Wave. *Index Score of 100 = No change between Baseline and Current Wave.

National Market Research. Brand Strength Monitor Summary Results — Spring 2011, Southern California.

Figure 4: *Patient Care Experience*

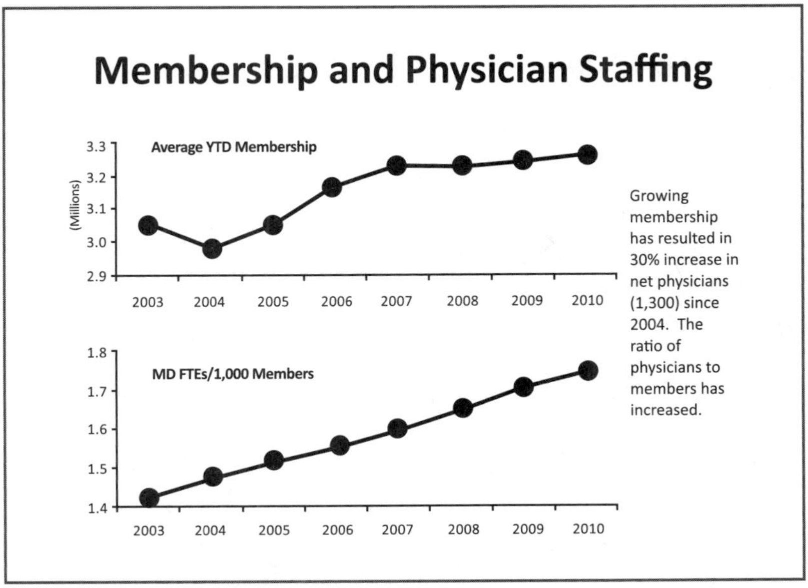

Figure 5: *Membership and Physician Staffing*

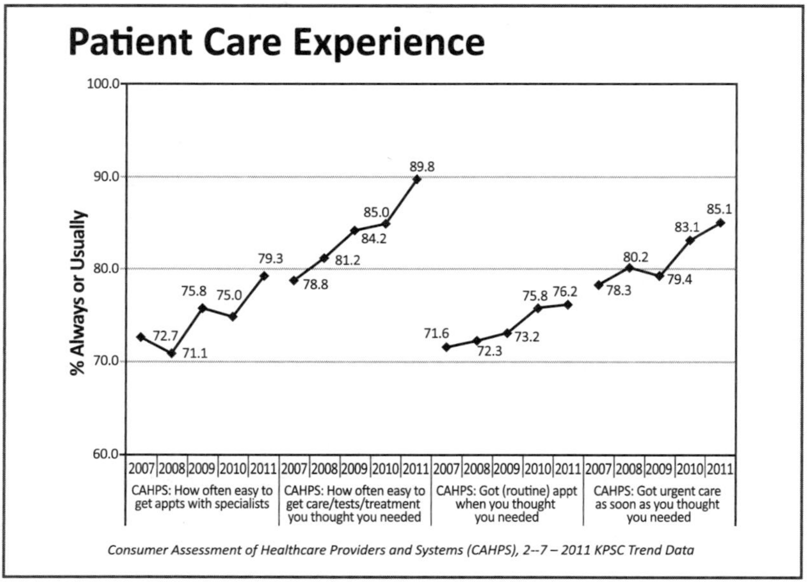

Figure 6: *Patient Care Experience*

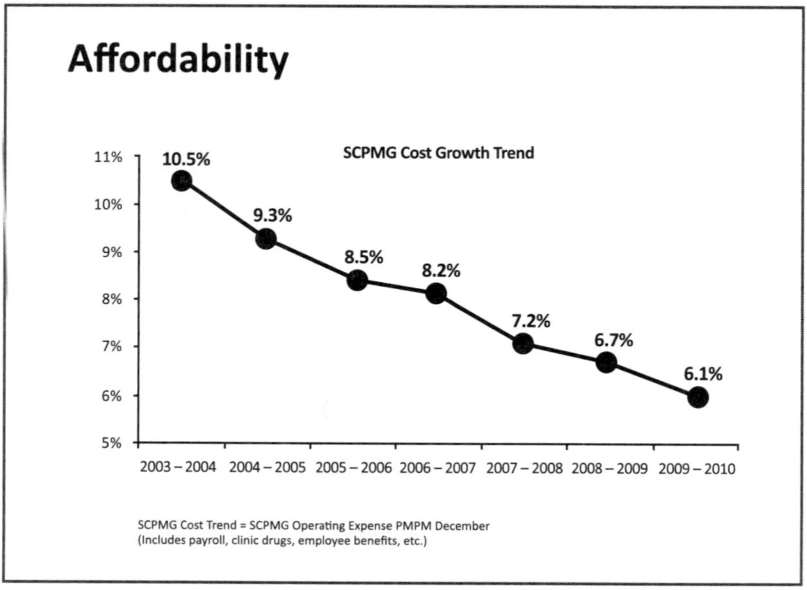

Figure 7: *Affordability*

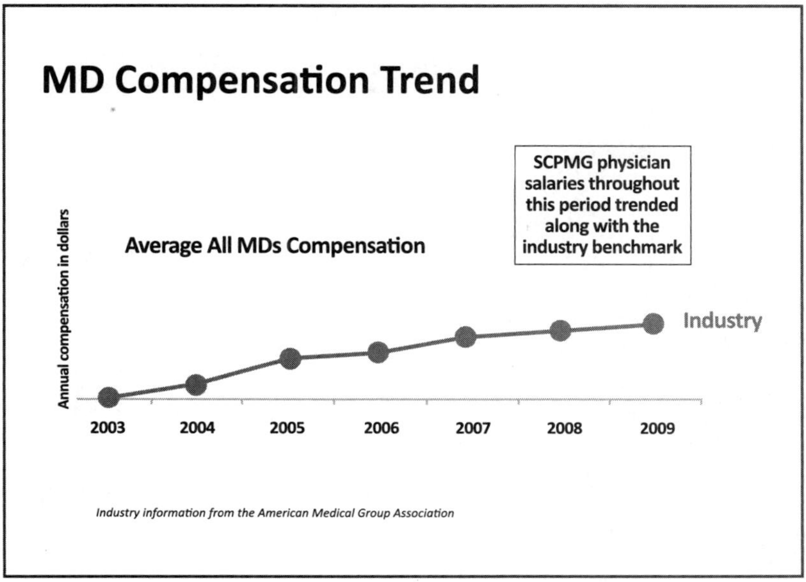

Figure 8: *MD Compensation Trend: Comparison with National Averages*

Acknowledgments*

In preparing this book, I drew on the perspectives and experiences of the following individuals. It includes individuals from SCPMG, Kaiser Permanente, the Coalition of Kaiser Permanente Unions, and other health systems. The efforts of many others at SCPMG and Kaiser Permanente were critical to the success we have had in improving value and outcomes at KPSC. In particular, I have had the pleasure of serving with an outstanding group of physicians on the Board of Directors of SCPMG, and in leadership capacities in SCPMG and the Southern California Region of Kaiser Foundation Health Plan and Hospitals. I express my deepest appreciation to all of you.

Fred Alamshaw, DO	Regional RUAT Chair Physician-in-Charge, Anaheim Hills Medical Office
John August	Executive Director, Coalition of Kaiser Permanente Unions
Julia Bae, MD	Area Medical Director, Kern County
John Brookey, MD	Assistant Medical Director, Quality & Risk Management
Maria Carrasco, MD	Regional Physician Coordinator, Culturally Responsive Care Family Medicine Physician, Baldwin Park
Ben Chu, MD	President, Southern California Region KFH/HP
Jack Cochran, MD	Executive Director, The Permanente Federation, LLC
Patricia De La Riva, MD	Pediatrics Physician, Woodland Hills Culturally Responsive Care Champion
James DeFontes, MD	Assistant Executive Medical Director Regional Director, Perioperative Services
Richard Dell, MD	Orthopedics Physician, Downey
Mark Eastman, MD	Family Medicine Physician, Riverside Physician Leader Proactive Care & Pathway to Proficiency

Titles were accurate as of December 2011.

Edward Ellison, MD	Executive Medical Director and Chairman of the Board, SCPMG
Howard Fullman, MD	Area Medical Director, West Los Angeles
Tad Funahashi, MD	Regional Chief, Orthopedic Surgery Assistant Area Medical Director, Orange County
George Halvorson	Chairman & Chief Executive Officer Kaiser Foundation Health Plan, Inc.
Patti Harvey	Senior Vice President, Quality and Risk Management Patient Care Services Clinical Operations Support
Joel Hyatt, MD	Assistant Medical Director, Regional Quality & Clinical Analysis
Michael Kanter, MD	Medical Director of Quality & Clinical Analysis
Marc Klau, MD	Regional Chief, Head & Neck Surgery
Alexander Lee, MD	Regional Chief, Gastroenterology
Gail Lindsay	Managing Director, Clinical Program Development
Russell Lo Bue	Clinical Director of Emergency Services
Ronald Loo, MD	Regional Chief, Urology
Robert Margolis, MD	Managing Partner & CEO of HealthCare Partners
Paul Minardi, MD	Medical Director of Operations
Alex Morales	Graphic Design, SCPMG Communications
Anita Moreno	Staff Specialist & Assistant to Medical Director of Operations
Brian Nguyen, MD	SCPMG Elected Board Member; Family Medicine Physician, South Bay; Physician Director of Clinical Strategic Goals Optimization
Debbie Ogawa	Management Consulting
Marilyn Owsley	Business Administrator of Finance, Systems & Consulting
Todd Sachs, MD	Chief of Surgery, West Los Angeles & SCPMG Elected Board Member
Denise Schaefer	Regional Director, Health Education
Jeffrey Selevan, MD	Medical Director of Business Management
Noreen Schob	Staff Specialist & Assistant to the Executive Medical Director, SCPMG
Joanne Schottinger, MD	Assistant Medical Director of Quality & Clinical Analysis

Mi Chelle Sorey	SCPMG Communications Manager
Nancy Spiegel	Manager, Permanente Leadership & Organizational Development
Steven Steinberg, MD	Chief of Service, Family Medicine-Panorama City
Kirk Tamaddon, MD	Director, Robotic Surgery Program
Kim Thai, MD	Regional Chief Physician, PM&R Regional Lead Physician, Pain Management
Bernard Tyson	Senior Vice President, Health Plan & Hospital Operations
Tom Williamson	Business Administrator of Operations
Teresa Wray, MD	Regional Chief, OB/GYN
Scott Young, MD	Occupational Medicine Physician, Northwest Permanente Member, Quality Management Committee

SCPMG Board of Directors

Medical Directors, Medical Group Administrators and Physicians of SCPMG

Health Plan and Hospital Leaders

Bibliography

Accountable Care Organization Learning Network. "ACO Model Principles." 2012. http://www.acolearningnetwork.org/why-we-exist/aco-model-principles.

Adamy, Janet. "WellPoint Shakes Up Hospital Payments." *Wall Street Journal*, May 16, 2011.

Agency for Healthcare Research and Quality. "CAHPS." n.d., https://www.cahps.ahrq.gov/content/cahpsOverview/OVER_Intro.asp.

AHRQ Health Care Innovations Exchange. "Service Delivery Innovation Profile: Capitated System Identifies, Screens, and Treats Osteoporosis Risks, Preventing Hip Fractures, Saving Lives, and Reducing Costs." June 27, 2011. http://www.innovations.ahrq.gov/content.aspx?id=2826.

Alliance of Community Health Plans. *Investing in Outcomes, Creating Value; ACHP Plans are Working to Reward Patient Outcomes*. n.d. http://www.achp.org/files.php?force&file=/ACHP_GroupHealth_CaseStudy_223348370.pdf.

Alliance of Community Health Plans. *Building Healthier Communities: Priority Health*. n.d. http://www.achp.org/files.php?force&file=/ACHP_PriorityHealth_CaseStudy_393651361.pdf.

Alliance of Community Health Plans. *Engaging Patients in their Health: HealthPartners*. n.d. http://www.achp.org/files.php?force&file=/ACHP_HealthPartners_CaseStudy_835434826.pdf.

Alliance of Community Health Plans. *Investing in Outcomes, Creating Value: Group Health*. n.d. http://www.achp.org/files.php?force&file=/ACHP_GroupHealth_CaseStudy_932428296.pdf.

American Academy of Family Physicians, American Academy of Pediatrics, American College of Physicians, and American Osteopathic Association. *Joint Principles of the Patient-Centered Medical Home.* March 2007. http://www.medicalhomeinfo.org/downloads/pdfs/jointstatement.pdf.

American Academy of Neurology. "AAN Practice Guidelines and Tools." 2011. http://www.aan.com/go/practice/guidelines.

American College of Radiology. "Practice Guidelines and Technical Standards."2011. http://www.acr.org/SecondaryMainMenuCategories/quality_safety/guidelines.aspx.

American Medical Association. "Benefits of an EMR,"October 24, 2006. http://www.ama-assn.org.

Anderson, Laurie M., Susan C. Scrimshaw, Mindy T. Fullilove, Jonathan E. Fielding, Jacques Normand, and the Task Force on Community Preventive Services. "Culturally Competent Healthcare Systems: A Systematic Review." *American Journal of Preventive Medicine* 24, no. 3S (2003): 68-79.

Andersson-Gäre, Boel, and Duncan Neuhauser. "The Health Care Quality Journey of Jönköping County Council, Sweden." *Q Manage Health Care* 16, no. 1 (2007): 2-9.

Andrews, Michelle. "Employers Roll Out Aggressive Wellness Programs." *US News & World Report* (October 25, 2007). http://health.usnews.com/health-news/health-plans/articles/2007/10/25/americas-best-health-plans.

Andrews, Michelle. "Many Workplace Clinics Offer Primary-Care Services." *Los Angeles Times*, May 25, 2011. http://articles.latimes.com/2011/may/25/health/la-he-workplace-clinics-20110525.

Appleby, Julie, and Sharon Silke Carty. "Ailing GM Looks to Scale Back Generous Health Benefits." *USA Today*, June 23, 2005. http://www.usatoday.com/money/autos/2005-06-22-gm-healthcare-usat_x.htm.

AT&T Healthcare. "AT&T Healthcare Community Online Physician Portal." 2012. http://www.corp.att.com/healthcare/physicianportal/

Audet, A.-M. J., Ramanathan Raju, Caroline M. Jacobs, J.F. Schick, and A.D. Aviles. "Transparency as a Pillar of a Quality and Safety Culture: The Experience of the New York City Health and Hospitals Corporation." *The Joint Commission Journal on Quality and Patient Safety* 34, no. 12 (2008): 707-712.

Bass, Frank. "AP: Pain Medicine Use Has Nearly Doubled." *Washington Post*, August 20, 2007. http://www.washingtonpost.com/wp-dyn/content/article/2007/08/20/AR2007082000147_pf.html.

Bate, Paul, and Glenn Robert. *Bringing User Experience to Healthcare Improvement: The Concepts, Methods and Practices of Experience-Based Design*. New York: Radcliffe Publishing, 2007.

Begley, Sharon. "The Best Medicine: Cutting Health Costs with Comparative Effectiveness Research." *Scientific American*, July 11, 2011, 50-55.

Berrington de González, Amy, Mahadevappa Mahesh, Kwang-Pyo Kim, Mythreyi Bhargavan, Rebecca Lewis, Fred Mettler, and Charles Land. "Projected Cancer Risks From Computed Tomographic Scans Performed in the United States in 2007." *Archives of Internal Medicine* 169, no. 22 (2009): 2071-2077. http://archinte.ama-assn.org/cgi/content/abstract/169/22/2071?ijkey=45e6d79523961652c2d366492e773a86a58e3913&keytype2=tf_ipsecsha.

Berry, Emily. "Medicare Advantage Plans Look for Physician Buy-In on Five-Star Rating System." *American Medical News*, October 31, 2011. http://www.ama-assn.org/amednews/m/2011/10/31/bsb1031.htm.

Berwick, Donald M., Thomas W. Nolan, and John Whittington. "The Triple Aim: Care, Health, and Cost," *Health Affairs* 27, no. 3 (2008): 759-769.

Blackmore, C. Craig, Robert S. Mecklenburg, and Gary S. Kaplan. "At Virginia Mason, Collaboration Among Providers, Employers, and Health Plans to Transform Care Cut Costs and Improved Quality." *Health Affairs* 30, no. 9,(2011): 1680-1687.

Blumberg, Jeremy M., Eric O. Kwon, T. Craig Cheetham, Fang Niu, Charles E. Shapiro, Judith Pacificar, Ronald K. Loo, Stephen G. Williams, and Gary W. Chien. "Early Development of Castrate Resistance Varies with Different Dosing Regimens of Luteinizing Hormone Releasing Hormone Agonist in Primary Hormonal Therapy for Prostate Cancer." *Urology* 77, no. 2 (2011): 412-416.

Bodenheimer, T., Mats Bojestig, and Goran Henriks. "Making Systemwide Improvements in Health Care: Lessons from Jönköping County, Sweden." *Q Manage Health Care* 16, no. 1 (2007): 10-15.

Broch, Jan. *Community-Based Transitional Care Improvement*. Colorado Foundation for Medical Care, n.d. http://www.acmq.org/natlconf/pdfs/brock.pdf.

Brooks, Rochelle, and Courtney Grotz. "Implementation of Electronic Medical Records: How Healthcare Providers are Managing the Challenges of Going Digital." *Journal of Business & Economics Research* 8, no. 6, (2010): 73-84.

"Business: Another American Way; Controlling Health-Care Costs." *The Economist* 395, no. 8680 (2010): 67.

Centers for Disease Control and Prevention . "Chronic Diseases: The Power to Prevent, the Call to Control." December 17, 2009. http://www.cdc.gov/chronicdisease/resources/publications/aag/chronic.htm#links.

Centers for Disease Control and Prevention. "Estimating Seasonal Influenza-Associated Deaths in the United States: CDC Study Confirms Variability of Flu." June 24, 2011. http://www.cdc.gov/flu/about/disease/us_flu-related_deaths.htm.

Centers for Medicare & Medicaid Services, *Medicare Physician Group Practice Demonstration*, Baltimore, July 2011. https://www.cms.gov/DemoProjectsEvalRpts/downloads/PGP_Fact_Sheet.pdf.

Chen, Jersey, Sharon-Lise T. Normand, Yun Wang, and Harlan M. Krumholz. "National and Regional Trends in Heart Failure Hospitalization and Mortality Rates for Medicare Beneficiaries, 1998-2008." *Journal of the American Medical Association* 306, no. 15 (2011): 1669-1678.

Christensen, Clayton M., Jerome H. Grossman, and Jason Hwang. *The Innovator's Prescription: A Disruptive Solution for Health Care*. New York: McGraw-Hill, 2008.

Christie, Les. "Number of People without Health Insurance Climbs." *CNNMoney*. September 13, 2011. http://money.cnn.com/2011/09/13/news/economy/census_bureau_health_insurance/index.htm.

Cleveland Clinic. *Facts and Figures*. November 23, 2010. http://my.clevelandclinic.org/Documents/About/facts-figures-2010.pdf.

Cleveland Clinic. "Benefits: Employee Wellness." n.d. http://my.clevelandclinic.org/careers/employee_wellness.aspx

Committee on Quality of Health Care in America, Institute of Medicine. *Crossing the Quality Chasm: A New Health System for the 21st Century*. Washington, DC: The National Academies Press, 2001.

Committees on Ways and Means, Energy and Commerce, and Education and Labor, *Affordable Health Care for America. Health Insurance Reform at a Glance: Implementation Timeline.* April 2, 2010. http://docs.house.gov/energycommerce/TIMELINE.pdf.

Commonwealth Fund. "States in Action: States' Role in Promoting Meaningful Use of Electronic Health Records." April/May 2011. http://www.commonwealthfund.org/Content/Newsletters/States-in-Action/2011/ May/April-May-2011/Feature/Feature.aspx.

Connolly, Ceci. "Cedars-Sinai Doctors Cling to Pen and Paper." *Washington Post*, March 21, 2005, A01.

Cosgrove, Delos M. "A Healthcare Model for the 21st Century." *Group Practice Journal* 60, no. 3 (2011): 11-15. http://my.clevelandclinic.org/Documents/redefining-healthcare/amga-mar-2011.pdf.

Coye, Molly Joel, Ateret Haselkorn, and Steven DeMello. "Remote Patient Management: Technology-Enabled Innovation and Evolving Business Models for Chronic Disease Care." Health Affairs 28, no 1 (2009): 126-135.

CVS/pharmacy minute clinic. "Vaccinations." Accessed September 13, 2012. http://www.minuteclinic.com/services/vaccination/?stateId=ca.

Davis, Brett J. "Improving Healthcare Outcomes through EBM." *Health Management Technology* 31, no. 10 (2010).

Davis, Dave, Mary Ann Thomson O'Brien, Nick Freemantle, Fredric M. Wolf, Paul Mazmanian, and Anne Taylor-Vaisey. "Impact of Formal Continuing Medical Education: Do Conferences, Workshops, Rounds, and Other Traditional Continuing Education Activities Change Physician Behavior or Health Care Outcomes?" *Journal of the American Medical Association* 282, no. 9 (1999): 867-874.

Davis, David A., Mary Ann Thomson, Andrew D. Oxman, and Brian R. Haynes. "Changing Physician Performance: A Systematic Review of the Effect of Continuing Medical Education Strategies." *Journal of the American Medical Association* 274, no. 9 (1995): 700-705.

Davis, Karen, Cathy Schoen, and Kristof Stremikis. *Mirror, Mirror on the Wall: How the Performance of the U.S. Healthcare System Compares Internationally*, 2010 Update. June 2010. http://www.commonwealthfund.org/Content/Publications/Fund-Reports/2010/Jun/Mirror-Mirror-Update.aspx?page=all

Davis, Karen. 2010 Annual Report President's Message: Realizing the Potential of Health Reform. Commonwealth Fund, 2011. http://www.commonwealthfund.org/~/media/Files/Annual%20Report/2010/2010_AR_Pres_Msg_1021.pdf.

Debley, Tom. "50 Years Ago: The Birth of Computers in KP Medicine." Kaiser Permanente: A History of Total Health, May 12, 2010. http://www.kaiserpermanentehistory.org/latest/50-years-ago-the-birth-of-computers-in-kp-medicine/.

Dentch, Courtney. "Actors Help Doctors-to-Be Rehearse their Bedside Manner." *Los Angeles Times*, May 15, 2006. http://articles.latimes.com/print/2006/may/15/entertainment/et-doctors15.

DeVol, Ross, and Armen Bedroussian. *An Unhealthy America: The Economic Burden of Chronic Disease; Charting a New Course to Save Lives and Increase Productivity and Economic Growth. Executive Summary and Research Findings.* Santa Monica, CA: Milken Institute, 2007. http://www.milkeninstitute.org/pdf/ES_ResearchFindings.pdf.

Deyell, Mark W., Christopher E. Buller, Louis H. Miller, Tracy Y. Wang, and David Dai. "Impact of national clinical guideline recommendations for revascularization of persistently occluded infarct-related arteries on clinical practice in the United States." *Archives of Internal Medicine*, July 11, 2008, E1-E8.

Dill, Michael J., and Edward S. Salsberg. *The Complexities of Physician Supply and Demand: Projections Through 2025*. Washington, DC: Association of American Medical Colleges, November 2008. https://members.aamc.org/eweb/upload/The%20Complexities%20of%20Physician%20Supply.pdf.

Doctor's Office Quality-Information Technology. Supporting Care Management: The Role of Electronic Health Record (HER) Systems. n.d. http://www.providersedge.com/ehdocs/ehr_articles/Supporting_Care_Management-the_Role_of_EHR_ Systems.pdf.

Donohue, Julie M., Marisa Cevasco, and Meredith B. Rosenthal. "A Decade of Direct-to-Consumer Advertising of Prescription Drugs." New England Journal of Medicine, 357 no. 7 (2007): 673-681.

Dooren, Jennifer Corbett. "Making Clinical Trials Less of a Tribulation: The Shift to Electronic Medical Records Makes it Easier to Recruit Patients – and Keep Them." *Wall Street Journal*, March 27, 2001.

Dopson, Sue, Louise FitzGerald, Ewan Ferlie, John Gabbay, and Louise Locock. "No Magic Targets! Changing Clinical Practice to Become More Evidence Based." *Healthcare Management Review* 27, no. 3 (2010): 35-47.

Druss, Benjamin G., Steven C. Marcus, Mark Olfson and Harold Alan Pincus. "The Most Expensive Medical Conditions in America." *Health Affairs* 21, no. 4(2002): 105-111.

Duffy, F. Daniel, and Eric S. Holmboe. "Self-Assessment in Lifelong Learning and Improving Performance in Practice." *Journal of the American Medical Association* 296, no. 9 (2006): 1137-1139.

Eckel, Robert H. "Nonsurgical Management of Obesity in Adults." *New England Journal of Medicine*, 358 (2008): 1941-1950. http://www.nejm.org/doi/full/10.1056/NEJMcp0801652#ref2.

Economist Intelligence Unit. *The Future of Healthcare in Europe*. 2011. http://www.janssenemea.com/sites/default/files/The%20Future%20Of%20Healthcare%20in%20Europe.pdf.

Edington, Dee W. *Zero Trends: Health as a Serious Economic Strategy*. Ann Arbor, MI: Health Management Research Center, 2009.

Eriksson, Margareta K., Lars Hagberg, Lars Lindholm, Eva-Britt Malmgren-Olsson, Jonas Österlind, and Mats Eliasson. "Quality of Life and Cost-Effectiveness of a 3-Year Trial of Lifestyle Intervention in Primary Health Care." *Archives of Internal Medicine* 170, no. 16 (2010): 1470-1479.

Eustis, Mark A. "Changing the Way We Deliver and Pay for Care." *Hospitals & Health Networks* 85, no. 5 (2011): 54.

Fairview. "Six Ways Fairview is Reforming Health Care." 2011. http://www.fairview.org/About/S_021596.

Fleming, Chris."U.S. Health Spending Projected to Grow 5.8 Percent Annually." *Health Affairs Blog*. July 28, 2011.http://healthaffairs.org/blog/2011/07/28/u-s-health-spending-projected-to-grow-5-8-percent-annually/.

Garber, Seth. Measuring Quality in Healthcare. January 2011. http://cpeehcc.com/presentations_2011/Measuring%20Quality%20in%20Health%20Care.pdf.

Gawande, Atul. "The Cost Conundrum: Annals of Medicine." *The New Yorker* 85 (June 1, 2009): 16.

Girion, Lisa, Scott Glover, and Doug Smith. "Drugs Now More Deadlier than Autos; Fueled by Highly Addictive Prescription Pain Medications, Fatal Overdoses have Surpassed Traffic Deaths Nationwide." *Los Angeles Times*, September 18, 2011, A.1.

Girion, Lisa."HMOs in Unstable Condition: Members Bolt to Other Plans; Preferred Provider Organizations Offer Greater Choice, and Employers Like Them Because They can Shift Rising Costs to Workers." *Los Angeles Times*, April 9, 2005.

Goodnough, Abby, and Kevin Sack. "Massachusetts Tries to Rein in its Health Costs." *New York Times*, October 17, 2011. http://www.nytimes.com/2011/10/18/us/massachusetts-tries-to-rein-in-its-health-care-cost.html?_r=1&hp=&adxnnl=1&adxnnlx=1318936316-am7TayNmhWBofWBf9OI8fw.

Gosfield, Alice G., and James L. Reinertsen. "The 100,000 Lives Campaign: Crystallizing Standards of Care for Hospitals.," *Health Affairs* 24, no. 6 (2005): 1560-1570.

Halvorson, George C., and George J. Isham. *Epidemic of Care: A Call for Safer, Better and More Accountable Health Care*. San Francisco: Jossey-Bass, 2003.

Hayes, Julia H. Daniel A. Ollendorf, Steven D. Pearson, Michael J. Barry, Philip W. Kantoff, Susan T. Stewart, Vibha Bhatnagar, Christopher J. Sweeney, James E. Stahl, and Pamela M. McMahon. "Active Surveillance Compared with Initial Treatment for Men with Low-Risk Prostate Cancer: A Decision Analysis." *Journal of the American Medical Association* 304, no 21 (2010): 2373-2380.

"HCAHPS Fact Sheet." May 2012. http://www.hcahpsonline.org/files/HCAHPS%20Fact%20Sheet%20May%202012.pdf.

Health Care Incentives. "Premise." 2010. http://www.prometheuspayment.org/node/7/#/1/1

Healthcare.gov."What's Changing and When: Improving Quality and Lowering Costs, Paying Physicians Based on Value Not Volume." n.d. Accessed September 12, 2012. http://www.healthcare.gov/law/timeline/index.html.

Helfand, Duke. "Providence, Doctors Join to Study and Improve Care, Cut Costs," *Los Angeles Times*, October 6, 2011, p. B3.

Hendee, William R., Gary J. Becker, James P. Borgstede, Jennifer Bosma, William J. Casarella, Beth A. Erickson, C. Douglas Maynard, James H. Thrall, and Paul E. Wallner. "Addressing Overutilization in Medical Imaging." *Radiology* 257 (October 2010): 240-245. http://radiology.rsna.org/content/257/1/240.full?sid=a9ea7752-595c-474c-831f-0f3509ac97ac.

House Committees on Ways and Means, Energy and Commerce, and Education and Labor. *Affordable Health Care for America. Health Insurance Reform at a Glance: Innovative Delivery System Reform*. March 20, 2010. http://docs.house.gov/energy commerce/DELIVERY_REFORM.pdf.
http://www.hschange.org/CONTENT/1166/.

Hyatt, Joel D., Timothy J. Batchelder, and Richard Wagner. "Improving Appropriate Prescription Drug Use to Best Practice: Supporting Evidence-Based Drug Use." *The Permanente Journal* 7, no. 2 (2003): 13-21.

Immunization Action Coalition. "Honor Roll for Patient Safety: Mandatory Influenza Vaccination for Healthcare Workers." August 30, 2012.
http://www.immunize.org/honor-roll/.

Indiana University Health. "Wellness Track." n.d. http://www.clarianemployeewellness.org/.

Institute for Culturally Competent Care. *Centers of Excellence in Culturally Competent Care – National Diversity.* Oakland, CA: Kaiser Permanente, n.d. http://info.kp.org/communitybenefit/assets/pdf/our_work/global/Centers_of_Excellece_Brochure.pdf.

Institute for Health Care Delivery Research. "Course Offerings." 2012. http://intermountainhealthcare.org/qualityandresearch/institute/courses/Pages/home.aspx.

Isabel Healthcare. "Individual Subscription Pricing for Isabel." 2012. http://www.isabelhealthcare.com/home/pricing_ind.

J.D. Power and Associates . "The Distinguished Hospital Program." 2012. http://businesscenter.jdpower.com/?f=/jdpacontent/CorpComm/Services/content/CertificationPrograms_Healthcare.htm.

Jaffe, Russell, Robert A. Nash, Richard Ash, Norman Schwartz, Robert Corish, Tammy Born, Harold Lazarus, and ASIMP Working Group on Healthcare Transparency. "Healthcare Transparency: Opportunity or Mirage." *Journal of Management Development* 25, no. 10 (2006): 981-995.

James, Brent C., and Lucy A. Savitz. "How Intermountain Trimmed Health Care Costs Through Robust Quality Improvement Efforts." *Health Affairs* 30, no. 6 (2011): 1185-1191.

Johns, Gary. "Presenteeism in the Workplace: A Review and Research Agenda." *Journal of Organizational Behavior* 31, no. 4 (2010): 519-542.

Jones, Thomas M. "Patient Participation in EHR Benefits." *Health Management Technology* 24.10, no. 64 (2003): 63.

Jung, Howard, Joseph Gleason, Jeff Slezak, Hetal Patel, Ronald Loo, and Steven Jacobsen. "Association of Hematuria on Microscopic Urinalysis and Risk of Urinary Tract Cancer." *Journal of Urology* 185 (May 2011): 1699.

Kaiser EDU.org . "U.S Health Care Costs." n.d. http://www.kaiseredu.org/Issue-Modules/US-Health-Care-Costs/Background-Brief.aspx.

Kaiser Family Foundation. *What's in the Stars? Quality Ratings of Medicare Advantage Plans, 2010.* Menlo Park, CA: Henry J. Kaiser Family Foundation, December 2009. http://www.kff.org/medicare/upload/8025.pdf.

Kaiser Permanente. "Kaiser Permanente OB Virtual Tours." 2011. http://xnet.kp.org/multimedia/obtours/.

Kanter, Michael, Osvaldo Martinez, Gail Lindsay, Kristen Andrews, and Cristine Denver. "Proactive Office Encounter: A Systematic Approach to Preventive and Chronic Care at Every Patient Encounter." *The Permanente Journal* 14, no. 3 (2010): 38-43.

Kaplan, Robert S., and Michael E. Porter. "How to Solve the Cost Crisis in Health Care." *Harvard Business Review* September 2011, http://hbr.org/2011/09/how-to-solve-the-cost-crisis-in-health-care/ar/1.

Kapoor, Mukul, C. "Evidence Based Medicine: Can Everything Be Evident?" *Annals of Cardiac Anaesthesia* 14, no. 1 (2011): 3-5.

Keehan, Sean P., Andrea M. Sisko, Christopher J. Truffer, John A. Poisal, Gigi A. Cuckler, Andrew J. Madison, Joseph M. Lizonitz, and Sheila D. Smith. "National Health Spending Projections through 2020: Economic Recovery and Reform Drive Faster Spending Growth." *Health Affairs* 30, no. 8 (2011): 1594-1605, http://content.healthaffairs.org/content/30/8/1594.full.

Kelley, Ed, Ernie Moy, Beth Kosiak, Dwight McNeill, Chunliu Zhan, Dan Stryer, and Carolyn Clancy. "Prevention Health Care Quality in America: Findings from the First National Healthcare Quality and Disparities Reports." *Preventing Chronic Disease*, July 2004. http://www.cdc.gov/pcd/issues/2004/jul/04_0031.htm.

Kim, So Young, Sung Gyeong Kim, Jong Hyock Park, and Eun Cheol Park. "Costs of Initial Cancer Care and Its Affecting Factors." *Journal of Preventive Medicine and Public Health* 42, no. 4 (2009): 243-250.

Kohn, Linda T., Janet M. Corrigan, and Molla S. Donaldson, eds. *To Err is Human: Building a Safer Health System*. Washington, DC: Institute of Medicine, 1999.

Labor Management Partnership – Coalition of Kaiser Permanente Unions + Kaiser Permanente. "What is a Unit-Based Team?" November 2, 2009. http://www.lmpartnership.org/learning/training/tools_ubt.html.

Labor Management Partnership – Coalition of Kaiser Permanente Unions + Kaiser Permanente. "UBT Basics." 2012. http://www.lmpartnership.org/ubt.

Lambrew, Jeanne M. "A Wellness Trust to Prioritize Disease Prevention." *Policy Brief Series* (Hamilton Project), 4 (2007): 1-8., http://www.brookings.edu/research/papers/2007/04/useconomics-lambrew.

Landro, Laura. "The Informed Patient: When a Doctor isn't Enough – Nurse Navigators Help Patients through Maze of Cancer-Treatment Decisions, Fears." *Wall Street Journal*, August 16, 2011.

Leape, Lucian L. "Transparency and Public Reporting are Essential for a Safe Healthcare System." Commonwealth Fund, March 27, 2010. http://www.commonwealthfund.org/Content/Publications/Perspectives-on-Health-Reform-Briefs/2010/Mar/ Transparency -and-Public-Reporting-Are-Essential-for-a-Safe-Health-Care-System .aspx.

Lohr, Steve. "A Hospital is Offering Digital Records," New York Times, April 6, 2009, B.3.

Lohr, Steve. "Big Medical Groups Begin Patient Data-Sharing Project." Bits (blog), *New York Times*, April 6, 2011. http://bits.blogs.nytimes.com/2011/04/06/big-medical-groups-begin-patient-data-sharing-project/#.

Longman, Phillip. *Best Care Anywhere: Why VA Health Care is Better than Yours*. San Francisco: Polipoint Press, 2007.

Loo, Ronald, Joel Whittaker, and Violeta Rabrenivich. "National Practice Recommendations for Hematuria: How to Evaluate in the Absence of Strong Evidence?" *The Permanente Journal* 13, no. 1 (2009): 37.

Lorig, Kate R., David S. Sobel, Anita L. Stewart, Byron William Brown, Jr., Albert Bandura, Philip Ritter, Virginia M. Gonzalez, Diana D. Laurent, and Halsted R. Holman. "Evidence Suggesting that a Chronic Disease Self-Management Program can Improve Health Status while Reducing Hospitalizations: A Randomized Trial." *Medical Care* 37, no. 1 (January, 1999): 5-14.

Mankin, Donald, Susan G. Cohen, and Tora K. Bikson. *Teams and Technology: Fulfilling the Promise of the New Organization.* Boston: Harvard Business School Press, 1996.

Marcille, John. "A Conversation with Michael Kanter, MD: Casting a Wider Net." *Managed Care*, June 2011. http://www.managedcaremag.com/archives/1106/1106.qna_kanter.html.

Martin, Anne B., David Lassman, Benjamin Washington, Aaron Catlin, and the National Health Expenditure Accounts Team. "Growth in US Health Spending Remained Slow in 2010; Health Share of Gross Domestic Product was Unchanged from 2009." *Health Affairs* 31, no. 1 (2012): 208-219, http://content.healthaffairs.org/content/31/1/208.full.

Mascia, Daniele, and Americo Cicchetti. "Physician Social Capital and the Reported Adoption of Evidence-Based Medicine: Exploring the Role of Structural Holes." *Social Science & Medicine* 72 (2011): 798-805.

Mazmanian, Paul E., and David A. Davis. "Continuing Medical Education and the Physician as a Learner: Guide to the Evidence." *Journal of the American Medical Association* 288, no. 9 (2002): 1057-1060.

McGlynn, Elizabeth A., Steven M. Asch, John Adams, Joan Keesey, Jennifer Hicks, Alison DeCristofaro, and Eve A. Kerr. "The Quality of Health Care Delivered to Adults in the United States." *New England Journal of Medicine* 348, no. 26 (2003): 2635-2645.

Medicare and Medicaid Programs; Electronic Health Record Incentive Program; Final Rule, 42 CFR parts 412, 413, 422 et al. July 28, 2010. http://edocket.access.gpo.gov/2010/pdf/2010-17207.pdf.

Medicare and Medicaid Programs; Electronic Health Record Incentive Program; Final Rule, 42 CFR parts 412, 413, 422 et al. (July 28, 2010). http://edocket.access.gpo.gov/2010/pdf/2010-17207.pdf.

Miller, David C., Cathryn Gust, Justin B. Dimick, Nancy Birkmeyer, Jonathan Skinner, and John D. Birkmeyer. "Large Variations in Medicare Payments for Surgery Highlight Savings Potential from Bundled Payment Programs." *Health Affairs* 30, no. 11 (2011): 2107-2115.

Mohrman, Susan Albers, and Arienne McCracken. "A Physician Turned Leader Commits to Building an Award Winning Organization." In *Lessons in Leadership: Learning from Real World Cases*, edited by Donald D. Warrick and Jens Mueller, 1-7. Chicago: Rossi – Smith, 2011.

Mohrman, Susan Albers, Susan G. Cohen, and Allan M. Mohrman, Jr. *Designing Team-Based Organizations: New Forms for Knowledge Work*. San Francisco: Jossey-Bass, 1995.

Morris, Tommy J., John Pajak, Frank Havlik, Jessica Kenyon, and Dean Calcagni. "Battlefield Medical Information System-Tactical (BMIST): The Application of Mobile Computing Technologies to Support Health Surveillance in the Department of Defense." *Telemedicine and e-Health* 12, no. 4 (2006): 409-416.

Mulcahy, Nick."Late-State Cancer Diagnoses are Common, Says CDC Report." *Medscape Medical News*, November 29, 2010, http://www.medscape.com/viewarticle/733259.

Myers, Sue, Richard W. Grant, Nancy E. Lugn, Beth Holbert, and Joseph C. Kvedar. "Impact of home-based monitoring on the care of patients with congestive heart failure." *Home Health Care Management & Practice* 18, no. 6 (2006): 444-451.

National Center for Chronic Disease Prevention and Health Promotion. *The Power of Prevention: Chronic Disease... The Public Health Challenge of the 21st Century*. 2009. http://www.cdc.gov/chronicdisease/pdf/2009-Power-of-Prevention.pdf.

National Committee for Quality Assurance. "What is HEDIS?" 2011. http://www.ncqa.org/tabid/187/Default.aspx.

Navarro, Ronald A., Denise Greene, Raoul Burchette, Tadashi Funahashi, and Richard Dell. "Minimizing Disparities in Osteoporosis Care of Minorities with an Electronic Medical Record Care Plan." *Clinical Orthopaedics and Related Research* 469, no 7 (2011).

NCQA. "Diabetes Recognition Program." 2011. http://www.ncqa.org/tabid/139/Default.aspx.

NCQA. "Multicultural Health Care Distinction." 2011. http://www.ncqa.org/tabid/1195/Default.aspx.

New York State Department of Health. "Transitional Care Resources.," n.d. http://www.health.state.ny.us/professionals/patients/discharge_planning/transitional_care_resources.htm.

Office of Minority Health. "National Standards on Culturally and Linguistically Appropriate Services." April 12, 2007. http://minorityhealth.hhs.gov/templates/browse.aspx?lvl=2&lvlID=15.

Okie, Susan. "A Flood of Opioids, a Rising Tide of Death." *New England Journal of Medicine* 262, no. 21 (2010): 1981-1985.

Østbye, Truls, Kimberly S. H. Yarnall, Katrina M. Krause, Kathryn I. Pollak, Margaret Gradison, and J. Lloyd Michener. Is There Time for Management of Patients with Chronic Diseases in Primary Care?" *Annals of Family Medicine* 3, no. 3 (2005): 209–14.

Ozminkowski, Ronald J., Ron Z. Goetzel, Feifei Wang, Teresa B. Gibson, David Shechter, Shirley Musich, Joel Bender, and Dee W. Edington. "The Savings Gained from Participation in Health Promotion Programs for Medicare Beneficiaries." *Journal of Occupational and Environmental Medicine* 48, no. 11 (2006): 1125-1132.

Palmetto Health. "Palmetto Health Nurse Navigators." n.d. Accessed September 12, 2012. http://www.palmettohealth.org/body.cfm?id=1008.

Pate, Russell R., Michael Pratt, Steven N. Blair, William L. Haskell, Caroline A. Macera, Claude Bouchard, David Buchner et al. "Physical Activity and Public Health: A Recommendation from the Centers for Disease Control and Prevention and the American College of Sports Medicine." *Journal of the American Medical Association* 273, no. 5 (1995): 402-407.

Patient Protection and Affordable Care Act. Pub. L. No. 111-148, 124 Stat. 119. 2010. http://www.gpo.gov/fdsys/pkg/PLAW-111publ148/pdf/PLAW-111publ148.pdf.

Patorno, Elisabetta, Rhonda L. Bohn, Peter M. Wahl, Jerry Avorn, Amanda R. Patrick, Jun Liu, and Sebastian Schneeweiss. "Anticonvulsant Medications and the Risk of Suicide, Attempted Suicide, or Violent Death." *Journal of the American Medical Association* 303, no. 14 (2010), http://jama.ama-assn.org/content/303/14/1401.

Perocchia, Rosemarie Slevin, Julie Keany Hodorowski, Laurie A. Williams, Julie Kornfeld, Nydia Lassalle Davis, MaryAnn Monroe, and Mary Anne Bright. "Patient-Centered Communication in Cancer Care: The Role of the NCI's Cancer Information Service." *Journal of Cancer Education* 26, no. 1 (2011): 36-43.

POLST. "How Advance Directives and Physician Orders for Life-Sustaining Treatment (POLST) Compare." 2008. http://www.ohsu.edu/polst/programs/POLSTvAD.htm.

Porter, Michael E. "A Strategy for Healthcare Reform: Toward a Value-Based System." *New England Journal of Medicine* 361, no. 2 (2009): 109-112.

Porter, Michael E. "What is Value in Healthcare?" New England Journal of Medicine 363, no. 26 (2010): 2477-2481.

Porter, Michael E., and Elizabeth Olmsted Teisberg. "How Physicians Can Change the Future of Healthcare." *Journal of the American Medical Association* 297, no. 10 (2007): 1103-1111.

Premier. "New Accountable Care Organization Collaboratives will Focus on Creating Healthier Communities." News release, May 20, 2010. http://www.premierinc.com/about/news/10-may/aco052010.jsp.

Rasouli, Tannaz. "HHS Announce Prevention and Public Health Funding through ACA." *Association of American Medical Colleges*, June 25, 2010. https://www.aamc.org/advocacy/washhigh/highlights2010/162644/hhs_announces_prevention_and_public_health_funding_through_aca.html.

Redberg, Rita F. "Cancer Risks and Radiation Exposure From Computed Tomographic Scans: How Can We Be Sure that the Benefits Outweigh the Risks?" *Archives of Internal Medicine* 169, no. 22 (2009): 2049-2050. http://archinte.ama-assn.org/cgi/content/full/169/22/2049?maxtoshow=&hits=10&RESULTFORMAT=&fulltext=overuse+CT+scans&searchid=1&FIRSTINDEX=0&resourcetype=HWCIT#REF-IED90030-2.

Rittenhouse, Diane R., Stephen M. Shortell, and Elliott S. Fisher. "Primary Care and Accountable Care – Two Essential Elements of Delivery-System Reform." *New England Journal of Medicine* 361 (2009): 2301-2303. http://www.nejm.org/doi/full/10.1056/NEJMp0909327.

Sackett, David L., and William M. C. Rosenberg. "The Need for Evidence-Based Medicine." *Journal of the Royal Society of Medicine* 99 (1995): 620-624.

Sackett, David L., William M. C. Rosenberg, J. A. Muir Gray, R. Brian Haynes, and W. Scott Richardson., "Evidence Based Medicine: What It Is and What It Isn't." *BMJ* 312, no. 71 (1996).

Safran, Charles. "Electronic Medical Records: A Decade of Experience." *Journal of the American Medical Association* 285, no. 13 (2001): 1766.

Sandman, David, and Anthony Kovner. "A Philanthropy Tackles Growth in Health Costs at the State Level." *Health Affairs* 29, no. 7 (2010): 1411-1414.

Schoen, Cathy, Robin Osborn, David Squires, Michelle Doty, Petra Rasmussen, Roz Pierson, and Sandra Applebaum. "A Survey Of Primary Care Doctors In Ten Countries Shows Progress In Use Of Health Information Technology, Less In Other Areas." *Health Affairs*, 31, no. 12 (2012): 2805-2816.

Shortell, Stephen M., Lawrence P. Casalino, and Elliott S. Fisher. "Achieving the Vision: Structural Change." In *Partners in Health: How Physicians and Hospitals Can Be Accountable Together*, edited by Francis J. Crosson and Laura A. Tollen, 46-71. San Francisco: Jossey-Bass, 2010.

Sinsky, Christine A., Thomas A. Sinsky, Debra Althaus, Joan Tranel, and Maggie Thiltgen. "'Core Teams': Nurse-Physician Partnerships Provide Patient-Centered Care at an Iowa Practice." *Health Affairs* 29, no. 5 (2010): 966-968.

Smedley, Brian D., Adrienne Y. Stith, and Alan R. Nelson, eds.; Committee on Understanding and Eliminating Racial and Ethnic Disparities in Health Care, Board on Health Sciences Policy, Institute of Medicine. *Unequal Treatment: Confronting Racial and Ethnic Disparities in Health Care.* Washington DC: The National Academies Press, 2003.

Smelcer, John B., Hal Miller-Jacobs, and Lyle Kantrovich. "Usability of Electronic Medical Records." *Journal of Usability Studies* 4, no. 2 (2009): 70-84.

Smith, Amy, and Tracey Ferriss. "Home Health Monitoring May Significantly Improve Blood Pressure Control, Kaiser Permanente Study Finds." News release, May 21, 2010. http://xnet.kp.org/newscenter/pressreleases/co/2010/052110telehealthstudy.html.

Smith, Robert C., Francesca C. Dwamena, Madhusudan Grover, John Coffey, and Richard M. Frankel. "Behaviorally Defined Patient-Centered Communication: A Narrative Review of the Literature." *Journal of General Internal Medicine* 26, no. 2 (2011): 185-191.

Snyder, Lisa Lopez. "Insights for Creating Culturally Competent Healthcare Programs in the Latino Community." *Diversity Factor* 16, no. 1 (2008): 35-41.

Sperl-Hillen, JoAnn M., Beth Averbeck, Kevin Palattao, Jerry Amundson, Heidi Ekstrom, Bill Rush, and Patrick O'Connor. "Outpatient EHR-Based Diabetes Clinical Decision Support that Works: Lessons Learned from Implementing Diabetes Wizard." *Diabetes Spectrum* 23, no. 3 (2010): 150-154.

State Medical Licensure Requirements and Statistics, 2012. Continuing Medical Education for Licensure Reregistration. 2012. http://www.ama-assn.org/resources/doc/med-ed-products/continuing-medical-education-licensure.pdf.

Stewart, Walter F., Judith A. Ricci, Elsbeth Chee, David Morganstein, and Richard Lipton. "Lost Productive Time and Cost Due to Common Pain Conditions in the US Workforce." *Journal of the American Medical Association*, 290, no. 18 (2003): 2443-2454.

Straus, Sharon E., and Finlay A. McAlister. "Evidence-Based Medicine: A Commentary on Common Criticisms." *CMAJ* 163, no. 7 (2000): 834-841.

Stremikis, Kristof, Karen Davis, and Stuart Guterman. "Healthcare Opinion Leaders' Views on Transparency and Pricing." Commonwealth Fund, October 25, 2010. http://www.commonwealthfund.org/Content/Publications/Data-Briefs/2010/Oct/Health-Care-Opinion-Leaders-Views-on-Transparency-and-Pricing.aspx.

Sutherland, Jason M., Elliott S. Fisher, and Jonathan S. Skinner. "Getting Past Denial – The High Cost of Health Care in the United States." *New England Journal of Medicine*, 361 (2009): 1227-1230. http://www.nejm.org/doi/full/10.1056/NEJMp0907172.

Terpeluk, Paul. "Opposing View: Why We Won't Hire Smokers." *USA Today*, January 29, 2012. http://www.usatoday.com/news/opinion/story/2012-01-29/Cleveland-Clinic-not-hiring-smokers/52873896/1.

The Cochrane Library. "About the Cochrane Library." 2012. http://www.thecochranelibrary.com/view/0/AboutTheCochraneLibrary.html.

The Joint Commission. "Core Measure Sets." 2012. http://www.jointcommission.org/core_measure_sets.aspx.

The Leapfrog Group. "About Leapfrog." 2012. http://www.leapfroggroup.org/about_us.

The World Bank. "GDP growth (annual %)." 2012. http://data.worldbank.org/indicator/NY.GDP.MKTP.KD.ZG.

Timmermans, Stefan, and Aaron Mauck, "The Promises and Pitfalls of Evidence-Based Medicine." *Health Affairs* 24, no. 1 (2005): 18-28.

Timmins, Nicholas, "System Upgrade. " FT.com, May 28, 2009. http://www.ft.com/intl/cms/s/0/990cebfe-498c-11de-9e19-00144feabdc0.html#axzz26Sww3Swx.

Timmins, Nicholas. "Reform of NHS Records Plan Saves 700m Pounds." *FT.com.* http://www.ft.com/intl/cms/s/0/785e2f70-bc41-11df-8c02-00144feab49a.html#axzz26Sww3Swx

Toossi, Mitra. "Labor Force Projections to 2012: The Graying of the US Workforce." *Monthly Labor Review* 127, no. 2 (2004), 37-57.

Towers Watson. Raising the Bar on Health Care: Moving Beyond Incremental Change. 2010. http://www.towerswatson.com/assets/pdf/1345/TW_15565_NBGH.pdf.

Towner, Steven. "Chronic Disease Management at Intermountain Healthcare." *Frontiers of Health Services Management,* 25, no. 2 (Winter 2008): 3-14.

Tu, Ha T., Ellyn R. Boukus, and Genna R. Cohen. *Workplace Clinics: A Sign of Growing Employer Interest in Wellness.* Washington, DC: Center for Studying Health System Change, December 2010.

Tushman, Michael L., and Charles A. O'Reilly III. *Winning Through Innovation: A Practical Guide to Leading Organizational Change and Renewal.* Boston: Harvard Business School Publishing, 2002.

U.S. Department of Commerce. *We the American Elderly.* September 1993. http://www.census.gov/apsd/wepeople/we-9.pdf.

U.S. National Library of Medicine. "Fact Sheet MEDLINE." January 26, 2011. http://www.nlm.nih.gov/pubs/factsheets/medline.html.

United Nations Development Programme. Human Development Report 2005. 2005. http://hdr.undp.org/en/media/HDR05_complete.pdf.

US Census Bureau. "Language Spoken at Home: 2000 (QT-P16)." http://factfinder2.census.gov/faces/tableservices/jsf/pages/productview.xhtml?pid=DEC_00_110S_QTP16&prodType=table.

Vesely, Rebecca R. "The Doctor Will See You Now... At Your Office: Workplace Clinics Making a Resurgence." *Modern Healthcare* 41, no 22 (2011): 24-25.

Welch, H. Gilbert, and William C. Black. "Overdiagnosis in Cancer." *Journal of the National Cancer Institute,* 102, no. 2 (2010): 605-613.

Wells, Susan J. "Navigating the Expanding Wellness Industry: When Choosing among Vendors in the Fast-Growing Wellness Market, First Assess your Needs." *HRMagazine* 56, no. 3 (2011): 45.

Wennberg, John. "Time to Tackle Unwarranted Variations in Practice." BMJ, March 17, 2011. http://www.bmj.com/content/342/bmj.d1513.full.

Wiley-Blackwell, "Hospital Readmission Studies: Influencing Factors Identified." *ScienceDaily,* October 13, 2010. http://www.sciencedaily.com/releases/2010/10/101013082813.htm.

Wilson, Bruce. "Continuing Medical Education Programs Being Placed Under Closer Scrutiny." *CMAJ* 182, no. 14 (2010): E683-E684.

Winslow, Ron, and Shirley S. Wang. "Heart Failure Puts Fewer in Hospital." *Wall Street Journal,* October 19, 2011.

World Health Organization. *Influenza (Seasonal),* Fact Sheet # 211. April 2009. http://www.who.int/mediacentre/factsheets/fs211/en/.

World Health Organization. *Obesity and Overweight*, Fact Sheet #311. May 2012. http://www.who.int/mediacentre/factsheets/fs311/en/index.html.

Wu, Shinyi, and Anthony Green. *Projection of Chronic Illness Prevalence and Cost Inflation.* Santa Monica, CA: RAND, October, 2000.

Yanovski, Susan Z., and Jack A. Yanovski. "Obesity Prevalence in the United States — Up, Down, or Sideways?" *New England Journal of Medicine*, 364 (2011): 987-989. http://healthpolicyandreform.nejm.org/?p=13941.

Yarnall, Kimberly S. H., Kathryn I. Pollak, Truls Østbye, Katrina M. Krause, and J. Lloyd Michener. "Primary Care: Is There Enough Time for Prevention?" *American Journal of Public Health* 93, no. 4 (2003): 635–41.

Zauber, Ann G., Sidney J. Winawer, Michael J. O'Brien, Iris Lansdorp-Vogelaar, Marjolein van Ballegooijen, Benjamin F. Hankey, Weiji Shi, John H. Bond, Melvin Schapiro, Joel F. Panish, Edward T. Stewart, and Jerome D. Waye. "Colonoscopic Polypectomy and Long-Term Prevention of Colorectal-Cancer Deaths." *New England Journal of Medicine* 366, no. 8 (2012): 687-696.

Zhou,Yi Yvonne, Michael H. Kanter, Jian J. Wang, and Terhilda Garrido. "Improved Quality at Kaiser Permanente Through E-Mail Between Physicians and Patients." *Health Affairs* 29, no. 7, (2010): 1370-1375.

Zigmond, Jessica. "Explosion in Scan Rates." *Modern Healthcare* 40, no. 8 (2010): 12.

Endnotes

PREFACE ENDNOTES

[1] Lisa Girion, "HMOs in Unstable Condition: Members Bolt to Other Plans; Preferred Provider Organizations Offer Greater Choice, and Employers Like Them Because They can Shift Rising Costs to Workers," *Los Angeles Times*, April 9, 2005.

[2] Karen Davis, Cathy Schoen, and Kristof Stremikis, *Mirror, Mirror on the Wall: How the Performance of the U.S. Healthcare System Compares Internationally*, 2010 Update (June 2010), http://www.commonwealthfund.org/Content/Publications/Fund-Reports/2010/Jun/Mirror-Mirror-Update.aspx?page=all.

CHAPTER 1 ENDNOTES

[1] Les Christie, "Number of People without Health Insurance Climbs," *CNNMoney* (September 13, 2011), http://money.cnn.com/2011/09/13/news/economy/census_bureau_health_insurance/index.htm.

[2] Towers Watson, *Raising the Bar on Health Care: Moving Beyond Incremental Change* (2010), http://www.towerswatson .com/assets/pdf/1345/TW_15565_NBGH.pdf; The World Bank, "GDP growth (annual %)," 2012, http://data.worldbank.org/indicator/NY.GDP.MKTP.KD.ZG.

[3] Sean P. Keehan et al., "National Health Spending Projections through 2020: Economic Recovery and Reform Drive Faster Spending Growth," *Health Affairs* 30, no. 8 (2011): 1594-1605, http://content.healthaffairs.org/content/30/8/1594.full; Anne B. Martin et al., "Growth in US Health Spending Remained Slow in 2010; Health Share of Gross Domestic Product was Unchanged from 2009," *Health Affairs* 31, no. 1 (2012): 208-219, http://content.healthaffairs.org/content/31/1/208.full.

[4] Martin et al., "Growth in US Health Spending Remained Slow in 2010; Health Share of Gross Domestic Product was Unchanged from 2009," 208-219; Chris Fleming, "U.S. Health Spending Projected to Grow 5.8 Percent Annually," *Health Affairs Blog*, July 28, 2011, http://healthaffairs.org/blog/2011/07/28/u-s-health-spending-projected-to-grow-5-8-percent-annually/.

[5] Karen Davis, *2010 Annual Report President's Message: Realizing the Potential of Health Reform* (Commonwealth Fund, 2011), http://www.commonwealthfund.org/~/media/Files/Annual%20Report/2010/2010_AR_Pres_Msg_1021.pdf.

[6] Julie Appleby and Sharon Silke Carty, "Ailing GM Looks to Scale Back Generous Health Benefits," *USA Today*, June 23, 2005, http://www.usatoday.com/money/autos/2005-06-22-gm-healthcare-usat_x.htm.

[7] Mitra Toossi, "Labor Force Projections to 2012: The Graying of the US Workforce," *Monthly Labor Review* 127, no. 2 (2004), 37-57.

[8] American Academy of Family Physicians, American Academy of Pediatrics, American College of Physicians, and American Osteopathic Association, *Joint Principles of the Patient-Centered Medical Home*, March 2007, http://www.medicalhomeinfo.org/downloads/pdfs/jointstatement.pdf.

[9] "Business: Another American Way; Controlling Health-Care Costs," *The Economist* 395, no. 8680 (2010): 67.

[10] Donald M. Berwick, Thomas W. Nolan, and John Whittington. "The Triple Aim: Care, Health, and Cost," *Health Affairs* 27, no. 3 (2008): 759-769.

[11] House Committees on Ways and Means, Energy and Commerce, and Education and Labor, Affordable Health Care for America. *Health Insurance Reform at a Glance: Innovative Delivery System Reform*, (March 20, 2010), http://docs.house.gov/energycommerce/DELIVERY_REFORM.pdf.

[12] Centers for Medicare & Medicaid Services, Medicare Physician Group Practice Demonstration, (Baltimore: July 2011), https://www.cms.gov/DemoProjectsEvalRpts/downloads/PGP_Fact_Sheet.pdf.

[13] Alliance of Community Health Plans, *Investing in Outcomes, Creating Value; ACHP Plans are Working to Reward Patient Outcomes* (n.d.), http://www.achp.org/files.php?force&file=/ACHP_GroupHealth_CaseStudy_223348370.pdf.

[14] Michael E. Porter, "What is Value in Healthcare?" *New England Journal of Medicine* 363, no. 26 (2010): 2477-2481.

[15] Committees on Ways and Means, Energy and Commerce, and Education and Labor, *Affordable Health Care for America. Health Insurance Reform at a Glance: Implementation Timeline* (April 2, 2010), http://docs.house.gov/energycommerce/TIMELINE.pdf.

[16] Abby Goodnough and Kevin Sack, "Massachusetts Tries to Rein in its Health Costs," *New York Times*, October 17, 2011, http://www.nytimes.com/2011/10/18/us/massachusetts-tries-to-rein-in-its-health-care-cost.html?_r=1&hp=&adxnnl=1&adxnnlx=1318936316-am7TayNmhWBofWBf9OI8fw.

[17] House Committees on Ways and Means, Energy and Commerce, and Education and Labor, *Affordable Health Care for America. Health Insurance Reform at a Glance: Innovative Delivery System Reform*, (March 20, 2010), http://docs.house.gov/energycommerce/DELIVERY_REFORM.pdf.

[18] United Nations Development Programme, *Human Development Report 2005* (2005), http://hdr.undp.org/en/media/HDR05_complete.pdf.

[19] Robert H. Eckel, "Nonsurgical Management of Obesity in Adults," *New England Journal of Medicine*, 358 (2008): 1941-1950, http://www.nejm.org/doi/full/10.1056/NEJMcp0801652#ref2.

[20] World Health Organization, *Obesity and Overweight*, Fact Sheet #311 (May 2012), http://www.who.int/mediacentre/factsheets/fs311/en/index.html.

[21] Russell R. Pate et al., "Physical Activity and Public Health: A Recommendation from the Centers for Disease Control and Prevention and the American College of Sports Medicine," *Journal of the American Medical Association* 273, no. 5 (1995): 402-407.

[22] Ron Winslow and Shirley S. Wang, "Heart Failure Puts Fewer in Hospital," *Wall Street Journal*, October 19, 2011. In addition, *The Wall Street Journal* article cites this study: Jersey Chen et al., "National and Regional Trends in Heart Failure Hospitalization and Mortality Rates for Medicare Beneficiaries, 1998-2008," *Journal of the American Medical Association* 306, no. 15 (2011): 1669-1678.

[23] Gary Johns, "Presenteeism in the Workplace: A Review and Research Agenda," *Journal of Organizational Behavior* 31, no. 4 (2010): 519-542.

[24] Susan J. Wells, "Navigating the Expanding Wellness Industry: When Choosing among Vendors in the Fast-Growing Wellness Market, First Assess your Needs," *HRMagazine* 56, no. 3 (2011): 45.

[25] Courtney Dentch, "Actors Help Doctors-to-Be Rehearse their Bedside Manner," *Los Angeles Times*, May 15, 2006, http://articles.latimes.com/print/2006/may/15/entertainment/et-doctors15.

[26] Robert C. Smith et al., "Behaviorally Defined Patient-Centered Communication: A Narrative Review of the Literature," *Journal of General Internal Medicine* 26, no. 2 (2011): 185-191.

[27] Rosemarie Slevin Perocchia et al., "Patient-Centered Communication in Cancer Care: The Role of the NCI's Cancer Information Service," *Journal of Cancer Education* 26, no. 1 (2011): 36-43.

[28] Julie M. Donohue, Marisa Cevasco, and Meredith B. Rosenthal, "A Decade of Direct-to-Consumer Advertising of Prescription Drugs," *New England Journal of Medicine*, 357 no. 7 (2007): 673-681.

[29] Medicare and Medicaid Programs; Electronic Health Record Incentive Program; Final Rule, 42 CFR parts 412, 413, 422 et al. (July 28, 2010), http://edocket.access.gpo.gov/2010/pdf/2010-17207.pdf.

[30] Steve Lohr, "Big Medical Groups Begin Patient Data-Sharing Project," *Bits* (blog), *New York Times*, April 6, 2011, http://bits.blogs.nytimes.com/2011/04/06/big-medical-groups-begin-patient-data-sharing-project/#.

[31] "What's Changing and When: Improving Quality and Lowering Costs, Paying Physicians Based on Value Not Volume," Healthcare.gov, n.d., accessed September 12, 2012, http://www.healthcare.gov/law/timeline/index.html.

[32] Committee on Quality of Health Care in America, Institute of Medicine. *Crossing the Quality Chasm: A New Health System for the 21st Century* (Washington, DC: The National Academies Press, 2001).

[33] George C. Halvorson and George J. Isham, *Epidemic of Care: A Call for Safer, Better and More Accountable Health Care* (San Francisco: Jossey-Bass, 2003), xxiii.

[34] Committee on Quality of Health Care in America, Institute of Medicine. *Crossing the Quality Chasm: A New Health System for the 21st Century.*

[35] "Palmetto Health Nurse Navigators," accessed September 12, 2012, http://www.palmettohealth.org/body.cfm?id=1008.

[36] Laura Landro, "The Informed Patient: When a Doctor isn't Enough - Nurse Navigators Help Patients through Maze of Cancer-Treatment Decisions, Fears," *Wall Street Journal*, August 16, 2011.

CHAPTER 2 ENDNOTES

[1] Elizabeth A. McGlynn et al., "The Quality of Health Care Delivered to Adults in the United States," *New England Journal of Medicine* 348, no. 26 (2003):2635-2645.

[2] Ed Kelley et al., "Prevention Health Care Quality in America: Findings from the First National Healthcare Quality and Disparities Reports," *Preventing Chronic Disease*, July 2004, http://www.cdc.gov/pcd/issues/2004/jul/04_0031.htm.

[3] Tannaz Rasouli, "HHS Announce Prevention and Public Health Funding through ACA," *Association of American Medical Colleges*, June 25, 2010, https://www.aamc.org/advocacy/washhigh/highlights2010/162644/hhs_announces_prevention_and_public_health_funding_through_aca.html

[4] Eckel, "Nonsurgical Management of Obesity in Adults," 1941-50.

[5] Eckel, "Nonsurgical Management of Obesity in Adults," 1941-50.

[6] Susan Z. Yanovski and Jack A. Yanovski, "Obesity Prevalence in the United States – Up, Down, or Sideways?" *New England Journal of Medicine*, 364 (2011): 987-989, http://healthpolicyandreform.nejm.org/?p=13941

[7] Alliance of Community Health Plans, *Building Healthier Communities: Priority Health* (n.d.), http://www.achp.org/files.php?force&file=/ACHP_PriorityHealth_CaseStudy_393651361.pdf.

[8] World Health Organization, *Influenza (Seasonal)*, Fact Sheet # 211 (April 2009), http://www.who.int/mediacentre/factsheets/fs211/en/.

[9] "Estimating Seasonal Influenza-Associated Deaths in the United States: CDC Study Confirms Variability of Flu," Centers for Disease Control and Prevention, June 24, 2011, http://www.cdc.gov/flu/about/disease/us_flu-related_deaths.htm.

[10] National Center for Chronic Disease Prevention and Health Promotion, *The Power of Prevention: Chronic Disease... The Public Health Challenge of the 21st Century* (2009), http://www.cdc.gov/chronicdisease/pdf/2009-Power-of-Prevention.pdf.

[11] "Chronic Diseases: The Power to Prevent, the Call to Control," Centers for Disease Control and Prevention, December 17, 2009, http://www.cdc.gov/chronicdisease/resources/publications/aag/chronic.htm#links.

[12] Jeanne M. Lambrew, "A Wellness Trust to Prioritize Disease Prevention," *Policy Brief Series* (Hamilton Project), 4 (2007): 1-8, http://www.brookings.edu/research/papers/2007/04/useconomics-lambrew.

[13] U.S. Department of Commerce, *We the American Elderly* (September 1993), http://www.census.gov/apsd/wepeople/we-9.pdf.

[14] Patient Protection and Affordable Care Act, Pub. L. No. 111-148, 124 Stat. 119 (2010), http://www.gpo.gov/fdsys/pkg/PLAW-111publ148/pdf/PLAW-111publ148.pdf.

[15] Economist Intelligence Unit, *The Future of Healthcare in Europe* (2011), http://www.janssen-emea.com/sites/default/files/The%20Future%20Of%20Healthcare%20in%20Europe.pdf.

[16] Alliance of Community Health Plans, *Engaging Patients in their Health: HealthPartners* (n.d.), http://www.achp.org/files.php?force&file=/ACHP_HealthPartners_CaseStudy_835434826.pdf.

[17] Steven Towner, "Chronic Disease Management at Intermountain Healthcare," *Frontiers of Health Services Management*, 25, no. 2 (Winter 2008): 3-14.

[18] Margareta K. Eriksson et al., "Quality of Life and Cost-Effectiveness of a 3-Year Trial of Lifestyle Intervention in Primary Health Care," *Archives of Internal Medicine* 170, no. 16 (2010): 1470-1479; Kate R. Lorig et al., "Evidence Suggesting that a Chronic Disease Self-Management Program can Improve Health Status while Reducing Hospitalizations: A Randomized Trial," *Medical Care* 37, no. 1 (January, 1999): 5-14.

[19] Linda T. Kohn, Janet M. Corrigan, and Molla S. Donaldson, eds., *To Err is Human: Building a Safer Health System* (Washington, DC: Institute of Medicine, 1999).

[20] "What is a Unit-Based Team?" Labor Management Partnership - Coalition of Kaiser Permanente Unions + Kaiser Permanente, November 2, 2009, http://www.lmpartnership.org/learning/training/tools_ubt.html

[21] Jane Broch, *Community-Based Transitional Care Improvement* (Colorado Foundation for Medical Care, n.d.), http://www.acmq.org/natlconf/pdfs/brock.pdf; see also "Transitional Care Resources," New York State Department of Health, n.d., http://www.health.state.ny.us/professionals/patients/discharge_planning/transitional_care_resources.htm, with resources for both patients and caregivers.

[22] Wiley-Blackwell, "Hospital Readmission Studies: Influencing Factors Identified." *ScienceDaily*, October 13, 2010, http://www.sciencedaily.com/releases/2010/10/101013082813.htm.

[23] Alliance of Community Health Plans, Investing in Outcomes, Creating Value: Group Health (n.d.), http://www.achp.org/files.php?force&file=/ACHP_GroupHealth_CaseStudy_932428296.pdf.

[24] Paul Terpeluk, "Opposing View: Why We Won't Hire Smokers," *USA Today*, January 29, 2012, http://www.usatoday.com/news/opinion/story/2012-01-29/Cleveland-Clinic-not-hiring-smokers/52873896/1.

[25] "Benefits: Employee Wellness," Cleveland Clinic, n.d., http://my.clevelandclinic.org/careers/employee_wellness.aspx

[26] Michelle Andrews, "Employers Roll Out Aggressive Wellness Programs," *US News & World Report* (October 25, 2007), http://health.usnews.com/health-news/health-plans/articles/2007/10/25/americas-best-health-plans; "Wellness Track," Indiana University Health, n.d., accessed September 13, 2012, http://www.clarianemployeewellness.org/.

[27] "Honor Roll for Patient Safety: Mandatory Influenza Vaccination for Healthcare Workers," Immunization Action Coalition, August 30, 2012, http://www.immunize.org/honor-roll/.

[28] Dee W. Edington, *Zero Trends: Health as a Serious Economic Strategy* (Ann Arbor, MI: Health Management Research Center, 2009), 66.

[29] Ronald J. Ozminkowski et al., "The Savings Gained from Participation in Health Promotion Programs for Medicare Beneficiaries," *Journal of Occupational and Environmental Medicine* 48, no. 11 (2006): 1125-1132.

CHAPTER 3 ENDNOTES

[1] Rosemarie Slevin Perocchia et al., "Patient-Centered Communication in Cancer Care: The Role of the NCI's Cancer Information Service," *Journal of Cancer Education*, 36-43.

[2] Paul Bate and Glenn Robert, *Bringing User Experience to Healthcare Improvement: The Concepts, Methods and Practices of Experience-Based Design* (New York: Radcliffe Publishing, 2007).

[3] "Vaccinations," CVS/pharmacy minute clinic, accessed September 13, 2012, http://www.minuteclinic.com/services/vaccination/?stateId=ca.

[4] Ha T. Tu, Ellyn R. Boukus, and Genna R. Cohen, *Workplace Clinics: A Sign of Growing Employer Interest in Wellness* (Washington, DC: Center for Studying Health System Change, December 2010), http://www.hschange.org/CONTENT/1166/.

[5] Rebecca R. Vesely, "The Doctor Will See You Now... At Your Office: Workplace Clinics Making a Resurgence," *Modern Healthcare* 41, no 22 (2011): 24-25.

[6] Michelle Andrews, "Many Workplace Clinics Offer Primary-Care Services," *Los Angeles Times*, May 25, 2011, http://articles.latimes.com/2011/may/25/health/la-he-workplace-clinics-20110525.

[7] Karen Davis et al., *Mirror, Mirror on the Wall: How the Performance of the U.S. Healthcare System Compares Internationally*, 2010 Update.

[8] "Kaiser Permanente OB Virtual Tours," Kaiser Permanente, 2011, http://xnet.kp.org/multimedia/obtours/.

[9] Laurie M. Anderson et al., "Culturally Competent Healthcare Systems: A Systematic Review," *American Journal of Preventive Medicine* 24, no. 3S (2003): 68-79.

[10] "Language Spoken at Home: 2000 (QT-P16)," US Census Bureau, http://factfinder2.census.gov/faces/tableservices/jsf/pages/productview.xhtml?pid=DEC_00_110S_QTP16&prodType=table

[11] "National Standards on Culturally and Linguistically Appropriate Services," Office of Minority Health, April 12, 2007, http://minorityhealth.hhs.gov/templates/browse.aspx?lvl=2&lvlID=15.

[12] John Marcille, "A Conversation with Michael Kanter, MD: Casting a Wider Net," *Managed Care*, June 2011, http://www.managedcaremag.com/archives/1106/1106.qna_kanter.html.

[13] Laurie M. Anderson et al., "Culturally Competent Healthcare Systems: A Systematic Review," 68-79.

[14] Lisa Lopez Snyder, "Insights for Creating Culturally Competent Healthcare Programs in the Latino Community," *Diversity Factor* 16, no. 1 (2008): 35-41.

[15] Institute for Culturally Competent Care, *Centers of Excellence in Culturally Competent Care - National Diversity* (Oakland, CA: Kaiser Permanente, n.d.), http://info.kp.org/communitybenefit/assets/pdf/our_work/global/Centers_of_Excellece_Brochure.pdf.

[16] Brian D. Smedley, Adrienne Y. Stith, and Alan R. Nelson, eds.; Committee on Understanding and Eliminating Racial and Ethnic Disparities in Health Care, Board on Health Sciences Policy, Institute of Medicine, *Unequal Treatment: Confronting Racial and Ethnic Disparities in Health Care* (Washington DC: The National Academies Press, 2003).

[17] Nick Mulcahy, "Late-State Cancer Diagnoses are Common, Says CDC Report," *Medscape Medical News*, November 29, 2010, http://www.medscape.com/viewarticle/733259; So Yung Kim et al., "Costs of Initial Cancer Care and Its Affecting Factors," *Journal of Preventive Medicine and Public Health* 42, no. 4 (2009): 243-250.

[18] Michael Kanter et al., "Proactive Office Encounter: A Systematic Approach to Preventive and Chronic Care at Every Patient Encounter," *The Permanente Journal* 14, no. 3 (2010): 38-43; Truls Østbye et al., "Is There Time for Management of Patients with Chronic Diseases in Primary Care?" *Annals of Family Medicine* 3, no. 3 (2005): 209–14; Kimberly S. H. Yarnall et al., "Primary Care: Is There Enough Time for Prevention?" *American Journal of Public Health* 93, no. 4 (2003): 635–41.

[19] Alliance of Community Health Plans, *Engaging Patients in their Health: HealthPartners* (n.d.), http://www.achp.org/files.php?force&file=/ACHP_HealthPartners_CaseStudy_835434826.pdf.

[20] Tommy J. Morris et al., "Battlefield Medical Information System-Tactical (BMIST): The Application of Mobile Computing Technologies to Support Health Surveillance in the Department of Defense," *Telemedicine and e-Health* 12, no. 4 (2006): 409-416.

[21] Molly Joel Coye, Ateret Haselkorn, and Steven DeMello, "Remote Patient Management: Technology-Enabled Innovation and Evolving Business Models for Chronic Disease Care," *Health Affairs* 28, no 1 (2009): 126-135.

[22] Amy Smith and Tracey Ferriss, "Home Health Monitoring May Significantly Improve Blood Pressure Control, Kaiser Permanente Study Finds," news release, May 21, 2010, http://xnet.kp.org/newscenter/pressreleases/co/2010/052110telehealthstudy.html.

[23] Julie M. Donohue et al., "A Decade of Direct-to-Consumer Advertising of Prescription Drugs," 673-681.

[24] H. Gilbert Welch and William C. Black, "Overdiagnosis in Cancer," *Journal of the National Cancer Institute*, 102, no. 2 (2010): 605-613.

[25] Julia H. Hayes et al., "Active Surveillance Compared with Initial Treatment for Men with Low-Risk Prostate Cancer: A Decision Analysis," Journal of the American Medical Association 304, no 21 (2010): 2373-2380.

[26] "How Advance Directives and Physician Orders for Life-Sustaining Treatment (POLST) Compare," POLST, 2008, http://www.ohsu.edu/polst/programs/POLSTvAD.htm.

CHAPTER 4 ENDNOTES

[1] Cathy Schoen et al., "A Survey Of Primary Care Doctors In Ten Countries Shows Progress In Use Of Health Information Technology, Less In Other Areas," *Health Affairs* 31, no. 12 (2012): 2805-2816.

[2] "Benefits of an EMR," American Medical Association, October 24, 2006, http://www.ama-assn.org.

[3] John B. Smelcer, Hal Miller-Jacobs, and Lyle Kantrovich, "Usability of Electronic Medical Records," *Journal of Usability Studies* 4, no. 2 (2009): 70-84.

[4] Nicholas Timmins, "System Upgrade," *FT.com*, May 28, 2009, http://www.ft.com/intl/cms/s/0/990cebfe-498c-11de-9e19-00144feabdc0.html#axzz26Sww3Swx.

[5] Timmins, "System Upgrade."

[6] Nicholas Timmins, "Reform of NHS Records Plan Saves 700m Pounds," *FT.com*, http://www.ft.com/intl/cms/s/0/785e2f70-bc41-11df-8c02-00144feab49a.html#axzz26Sww3Swx.

[7] John B. Smelcer, "Usability of Electronic Medical Records."

[8] Ceci Connolly, "Cedars-Sinai Doctors Cling to Pen and Paper," *Washington Post*, March 21, 2005, A01.

[9] "States in Action: States' Role in Promoting Meaningful Use of Electronic Health Records," Commonwealth Fund, April/May 2011, http://www.commonwealthfund.org/Content/Newsletters/States-in-Action/2011/May/April-May-2011/Feature/Feature.aspx.

[10] Medicare and Medicaid Programs; Electronic Health Record Incentive Program; Final Rule, 42 CFR parts 412, 413, 422 et al. (July 28, 2010), http://edocket.access.gpo.gov/2010/pdf/2010-17207.pdf.

[11] Rochelle Brooks and Courtney Grotz, "Implementation of Electronic Medical Records: How Healthcare Providers are Managing the Challenges of Going Digital," *Journal of Business & Economics Research* 8, no. 6, (2010): 73-84.

[12] Steve Lohr, "A Hospital is Offering Digital Records," *New York Times*, April 6, 2009, B.3.

[13] Charles Safran, "Electronic Medical Records: A Decade of Experience," *Journal of the American Medical Association* 285, no. 13 (2001): 1766.

[14] Doctor's Office Quality-Information Technology, *Supporting Care Management: The Role of Electronic Health Record (HER) Systems*, (n.d.), http://www.providersedge.com/ehdocs/ehr_articles/Supporting_Care_Management-the_Role_of_EHR_Systems.pdf.

[15] Thomas M. Jones, "Patient Participation in EHR Benefits," *Health Management Technology* 24.10, no. 64 (2003): 63.

[16] Yi Yvonne Zhou et al., "Improved Quality at Kaiser Permanente Through E-Mail Between Physicians and Patients," *Health Affairs* 29, no. 7, (2010): 1370-1375.

[17] Jennifer Corbett Dooren, "Making Clinical Trials Less of a Tribulation: The Shift to Electronic Medical Records Makes it Easier to Recruit Patients - and Keep Them," *Wall Street Journal*, March 27, 2001.

[18] Sharon Begley, "The Best Medicine: Cutting Health Costs with Comparative Effectiveness Research," Scientific American, July 11, 2011, 50-55.

[19] Sharon Begley, "The Best Medicine: Cutting Health Costs with Comparative Effectiveness Research," 50-55.

[20] Sue Myers et al., "Impact of home-based monitoring on the care of patients with congestive heart failure," *Home Health Care Management & Practice* 18, no. 6 (2006): 444-451.

CHAPTER 5 ENDNOTES

[1] Seth Garber, *Measuring Quality in Healthcare* (January 2011), http://cpeehcc.com/presentations_2011/Measuring%20Quality%20in%20Health%20Care.pdf; "What is HEDIS?" National Committee for Quality Assurance, 2011, http://www.ncqa.org/tabid/187/Default.aspx.

[2] Janet Adamy, "WellPoint Shakes Up Hospital Payments," *Wall Street Journal*, May 16, 2011.

[3] "What is HEDIS?" National Committee for Quality Assurance.

[4] "Core Measure Sets," The Joint Commission, 2012, http://www.jointcommission.org/core_measure_sets.aspx.

[5] Kaiser Family Foundation, *What's in the Stars? Quality Ratings of Medicare Advantage Plans*, 2010 (Menlo Park, CA: Henry J. Kaiser Family Foundation, December 2009), http://www.kff.org/medicare/upload/8025.pdf.

[6] "Premise," Health Care Incentives, 2010, http://www.prometheuspayment.org/node/7/#/1/1.

[7] "About Leapfrog," The Leapfrog Group, 2012, http://www.leapfroggroup.org/about_us.

[8] "HCAHPS Fact Sheet," May 2012, http://www.hcahpsonline.org/files/HCAHPS%20Fact%20Sheet%20May%202012.pdf.

[9] "The Distinguished Hospital Program," J.D. Power and Associates, 2012, http://businesscenter.jdpower.com/?f=/jdpacontent/CorpComm/Services/content/CertificationPrograms_Healthcare.htm.

[10] "Multicultural Health Care Distinction," NCQA, 2011, http://www.ncqa.org/tabid/1195/Default.aspx.

[11] "CAHPS," Agency for Healthcare Research and Quality, n.d., https://www.cahps.ahrq.gov/content/cahpsOverview/OVER_Intro.asp.

[12] See A-M. J. Audet et al., "Transparency as a Pillar of a Quality and Safety Culture: The Experience of the New York City Health and Hospitals Corporation," *The Joint Commission Journal on Quality and Patient Safety* 34, no. 12 (2008): 707-712, which discusses these categories of transparency as stages of implementation.

[13] Michael E. Porter, "A Strategy for Healthcare Reform: Toward a Value-Based System," *New England Journal of Medicine* 361, no. 2 (2009): 109-112. Kristof Stremikis, Karen Davis, and Stuart Guterman, "Healthcare Opinion Leaders' Views on Transparency and Pricing," Commonwealth Fund, October 25, 2010, http://www.commonwealthfund.org/Content/Publications/Data-Briefs/2010/Oct/Health-Care-Opinion-Leaders-Views-on-Transparency-and-Pricing.aspx. Russell Jaffe et al., "Healthcare Transparency: Opportunity or Mirage," *Journal of Management Development* 25, no. 10 (2006): 981-995.

[14] Lucian L. Leape, "Transparency and Public Reporting are Essential for a Safe Healthcare System," Commonwealth Fund, March 27, 2010, http://www.commonwealthfund.org/Content/Publications/Perspectives-on-Health-Reform-Briefs/2010/Mar/Transparency-and-Public-Reporting-Are-Essential-for-a-Safe-Health-Care-System.aspx.

[15] Committee on Quality of Health Care in America, Institute of Medicine. *Crossing the Quality Chasm: A New Health System for the 21st Century.*

[16] Michael E. Porter and Elizabeth Olmsted Teisberg, "How Physicians Can Change the Future of Healthcare," *Journal of the American Medical Association* 297, no. 10 (2007): 1103-1111.

[17] David C. Miller et al., "Large Variations in Medicare Payments for Surgery Highlight Savings Potential from Bundled Payment Programs," *Health Affairs* 30, no. 11 (2011): 2107-2115.

[18] Robert S. Kaplan and Michael E. Porter, "How to Solve the Cost Crisis in Health Care," *Harvard Business Review* September 2011, http://hbr.org/2011/09/how-to-solve-the-cost-crisis-in-health-care/ar/1

[19] Robert S. Kaplan and Michael E. Porter, "How to Solve the Cost Crisis in Health Care."

[20] Joel D. Hyatt, Timothy J. Batchelder, and Richard Wagner, "Improving Appropriate Prescription Drug Use to Best Practice: Supporting Evidence-Based Drug Use," *The Permanente Journal* 7, no. 2 (2003): 13-21.

[21] Susan Okie, "A Flood of Opioids, a Rising Tide of Death," *New England Journal of Medicine* 262, no. 21 (2010): 1981-1985.

[22] Lisa Girion, Scott Glover, and Doug Smith, "Drugs Now More Deadlier than Autos; Fueled by Highly Addictive Prescription Pain Medications, Fatal Overdoses have Surpassed Traffic Deaths Nationwide," *Los Angeles Times*, September 18, 2011, A.1.

[23] Linda T. Kohn et al., eds., *To Err is Human: Building a Safer Health System*; Alice G. Gosfield and James L. Reinertsen, "The 100,000 Lives Campaign: Crystallizing Standards of Care for Hospitals," *Health Affairs* 24, no. 6 (2005): 1560-1570.

[24] Emily Berry, "Medicare Advantage Plans Look for Physician Buy-In on Five-Star Rating System," *American Medical News*, October 31, 2011, http://www.ama-assn.org/amednews/m/2011/10/31/bsb1031.htm.

[25] Ann G. Zauber et al., "Colonoscopic Polypectomy and Long-Term Prevention of Colorectal-Cancer Deaths," *New England Journal of Medicine* 366, no. 8 (2012): 687-696.

[26] "Diabetes Recognition Program," NCQA, 2011, http://www.ncqa.org/tabid/139/Default.aspx.

CHAPTER 6 ENDNOTES

[1] Elizabeth A. McGlynn et al., "The Quality of Health Care Delivered to Adults in the United States," *New England Journal of Medicine* 348 (2003): 2635-2645.

[2] Mark W. Deyell et al., "Impact of national clinical guideline recommendations for revascularization of persistently occluded infarct-related arteries on clinical practice in the United States," *Archives of Internal Medicine*, July 11, 2008, E1-E8.

[3] Jason M. Sutherland, Elliott S. Fisher, and Jonathan S. Skinner, "Getting Past Denial - The High Cost of Health Care in the United States," *New England Journal of Medicine*, 361 (2009): 1227-1230, http://www.nejm.org/doi/full/10.1056/NEJMp0907172.

[4] Atul Gawande, "The Cost Conundrum: Annals of Medicine," *The New Yorker* 85 (June 1, 2009): 16.

[5] Sue Dopson et al., "No Magic Targets! Changing Clinical Practice to Become More Evidence Based," *Healthcare Management Review* 27, no. 3 (2010): 35-47.

[6] "Fact Sheet MEDLINE," U.S. National Library of Medicine, January 26, 2011, http://www.nlm.nih.gov/pubs/factsheets/medline.html.

[7] "About the Cochrane Library," The Cochrane Library, 2012, http://www.thecochranelibrary.com/view/0/AboutTheCochraneLibrary.html.

[8] "AAN practice guidelines and tools," American Academy of Neurology, 2011, http://www.aan.com/go/practice/guidelines.

[9] "Practice Guidelines and Technical Standards," American College of Radiology, 2011, http://www.acr.org/SecondaryMainMenuCategories/quality_safety/guidelines.aspx.

[10] Duke Helfand, "Providence, Doctors Join to Study and Improve Care, Cut Costs," *Los Angeles Times*, October 6, 2011, p. B3.

[11] Jeremy M. Blumberg et al., "Early Development of Castrate Resistance Varies with Different Dosing Regimens of Luteinizing Hormone Releasing Hormone Agonist in Primary Hormonal Therapy for Prostate Cancer," *Urology* 77, no. 2 (2011): 412-416.

[12] Elisabetta Patorno et al., "Anticonvulsant Medications and the Risk of Suicide, Attempted Suicide, or Violent Death," *Journal of the American Medical Association* 303, no. 14 (2010), http://jama.ama-assn.org/content/303/14/1401.

[13] Frank, Bass, "AP: Pain Medicine Use Has Nearly Doubled," *Washington Post*, August 20, 2007, http://www.washingtonpost.com/wp-dyn/content/article/2007/08/20/AR2007082000147_pf.html.

[14] David L. Sackett et al., "Evidence Based Medicine: What It Is and What It Isn't," *BMJ* 312, no. 71 (1996).

[15] Stefan Timmermans and Aaron Mauck, "The Promises and Pitfalls of Evidence-Based Medicine," *Health Affairs* 24, no. 1 (2005): 18-28.

[16] Mukul C. Kapoor, "Evidence Based Medicine: Can Everything Be Evident?" *Annals of Cardiac Anaesthesia* 14, no. 1 (2011): 3-5.

[17] Daniele Mascia and Americo Cicchetti, "Physician Social Capital and the Reported Adoption of Evidence-Based Medicine: Exploring the Role of Structural Holes," *Social Science & Medicine* 72 (2011): 798-805.

[18] Brett J. Davis, "Improving Healthcare Outcomes through EBM," *Health Management Technology* 31, no. 10 (2010).

[19] David L. Sackett and William M. C. Rosenberg, "The Need for Evidence-Based Medicine," *Journal of the Royal Society of Medicine* 99 (1995): 620-624.

[20] *Continuing Medical Education for Licensure Reregistration*, State Medical Licensure Requirements and Statistics, 2012, http://www.ama-assn.org/resources/doc/med-ed-products/continuing-medical-education-licensure.pdf.

[21] Bruce Wilson, "Continuing Medical Education Programs Being Placed Under Closer Scrutiny," *CMAJ* 182, no. 14 (2010): E683-E684.

[22] David A. Davis et al., "Changing Physician Performance: A Systematic Review of the Effect of Continuing Medical Education Strategies," *Journal of the American Medical Association* 274, no. 9 (1995): 700-705.

[23] Dave Davis et al., "Impact of Formal Continuing Medical Education: Do Conferences, Workshops, Rounds, and Other Traditional Continuing Education Activities Change Physician Behavior or Health Care Outcomes?" *Journal of the American Medical Association* 282, no. 9 (1999): 867-874.

[24] F. Daniel Duffy and Eric S. Holmboe, "Self-Assessment in Lifelong Learning and Improving Performance in Practice," *Journal of the American Medical Association* 296, no. 9 (2006): 1137-1139; Paul E. Mazmanian and David A. Davis, "Continuing Medical Education and the Physician as a Learner: Guide to the Evidence," *Journal of the American Medical Association* 288, no. 9 (2002): 1057-1060.

[25] Sharon E. Straus, and Finlay A. McAlister, "Evidence-Based Medicine: A Commentary on Common Criticisms," *CMAJ* 163, no. 7 (2000): 834-841.

[26] JoAnn M. Sperl-Hillen et al., "Outpatient EHR-Based Diabetes Clinical Decision Support that Works: Lessons Learned from Implementing Diabetes Wizard," *Diabetes Spectrum* 23, no. 3 (2010): 150-154.

[27] "AT&T Healthcare Community Online Physician Portal," AT&T Healthcare, 2012, http://www.corp.att.com/healthcare/physicianportal/.

[28] "Individual Subscription Pricing for Isabel," Isabel Healthcare, 2012, http://www.isabelhealthcare.com/home/pricing_ind.

CHAPTER 7 ENDNOTES

[1] Michael E. Porter, "What is Value in Health Care?" *New England Journal of Medicine* 363, no. 26 (2010): 2477-2481.

[2] Tom Debley, "50 Years Ago: The Birth of Computers in KP Medicine," Kaiser Permanente: A History of Total Health, May 12, 2010, http://www.kaiserpermanentehistory.org/latest/50-years-ago-the-birth-of-computers-in-kp-medicine/.

[3] "U.S Health Care Costs," Kaiser EDU.org, n.d., http://www.kaiseredu.org/Issue-Modules/US-Health-Care-Costs/Background-Brief.aspx.

[4] Ross DeVol and Armen Bedroussian, *An Unhealthy America: The Economic Burden of Chronic Disease; Charting a New Course to Save Lives and Increase Productivity and Economic Growth. Executive Summary and Research Findings* (Santa Monica, CA: Milken Institute, 2007), http://www.milkeninstitute.org/pdf/ES_ResearchFindings.pdf.

[5] Shinyi Wu and Anthony Green, *Projection of Chronic Illness Prevalence and Cost Inflation* (Santa Monica, CA: RAND, October, 2000).

[6] Ronald A. Navarro et al., "Minimizing Disparities in Osteoporosis Care of Minorities with an Electronic Medical Record Care Plan," *Clinical Orthopaedics and Related Research* 469, no 7 (2011).

[7] Navarro et al., "Minimizing Disparities in Osteoporosis Care of Minorities with an Electronic Medical Record Care Plan."

[8] "Service Delivery Innovation Profile: Capitated System Identifies, Screens, and Treats Osteoporosis Risks, Preventing Hip Fractures, Saving Lives, and Reducing Costs," AHRQ Health Care Innovations Exchange, June 27, 2011, http://www.innovations.ahrq.gov/content.aspx?id=2826.

[9] Walter F. Stewart et al., "Lost Productive Time and Cost Due to Common Pain Conditions in the US Workforce," *Journal of the American Medical Association*, 290, no. 18 (2003): 2443-2454; Benjamin G. Druss et al., "The Most Expensive Medical Conditions in America," Health Affairs 21, no. 4(2002): 105-111.

[10] John Wennberg, "Time to Tackle Unwarranted Variations in Practice," *BMJ*, March 17, 2011, http://www.bmj.com/content/342/bmj.d1513.full.

[11] David Sandman and Anthony Kovner, "A Philanthropy Tackles Growth in Health Costs at the State Level," *Health Affairs* 29, no. 7 (2010): 1411-1414.

[12] Mark A. Eustis, "Changing the Way We Deliver and Pay for Care," *Hospitals & Health Networks* 85, no. 5 (2011): 54; "Six Ways Fairview is Reforming Health Care," Fairview, 2011, http://www.fairview.org/About/S_021596.

[13] Porter, "What is Value in Health Care?"; Berwick, Nolan, and Whittington. "The Triple Aim: Care, Health, and Cost"; Diane R. Rittenhouse, Stephen M. Shortell, and Elliott S. Fisher, "Primary Care and Accountable Care – Two Essential Elements of Delivery-System Reform," *New England Journal of Medicine* 361 (2009): 2301-2303, http://www.nejm.org/doi/full/10.1056/NEJMp0909327.

[14] Clayton M. Christensen, Jerome H. Grossman, and Jason Hwang, *The Innovator's Prescription: A Disruptive Solution for Health Care* (New York: McGraw-Hill, 2008).

[15] Christensen, Grossman, and Hwang, *The Innovator's Prescription: A Disruptive Solution for Health Care.*

CHAPTER 8 ENDNOTES

[1] Patient Protection and Affordable Care Act, Pub. L. No. 111-148, 124 Stat. 119 (Section 3022), (2010).

[2] Premier, "New Accountable Care Organization Collaboratives will Focus on Creating Healthier Communities," news release, May 20, 2010, http://www.premierinc.com/about/news/10-may/aco052010.jsp; "ACO Model Principles, "Accountable Care Organization Learning Network, 2012, http://www.acolearningnetwork.org/why-we-exist/aco-model- principles.

[3] American Academy of Family Physicians, American Academy of Pediatrics, American College of Physicians, and American Osteopathic Association, *Joint Principles of the Patient-Centered Medical Home*.

[4] Delos M. Cosgrove, "A Healthcare Model for the 21st Century," *Group Practice Journal* 60, no. 3 (2011): 11-15, http://my.clevelandclinic.org/Documents/redefining-healthcare/amga-mar-2011.pdf.

[5] C. Craig Blackmore, Robert S. Mecklenburg, and Gary S. Kaplan, "At Virginia Mason, Collaboration Among Providers, Employers, and Health Plans to Transform Care Cut Costs and Improved Quality," *Health Affairs* 30, no. 9,(2011): 1680-1687.

[6] Donald Mankin, Susan G. Cohen, and Tora K. Bikson, Teams and Technology: *Fulfilling the Promise of the New Organization* (Boston: Harvard Business School Press, 1996).

[7] Mankin, Cohen, and Bikson, *Teams and Technology*.

[8] Michael J. Dill and Edward S. Salsberg, *The Complexities of Physician Supply and Demand: Projections Through 2025* (Washington, DC: Association of American Medical Colleges, November 2008), https://members.aamc.org/eweb/upload/The%20Complexities%20of%20Physician%20Supply.pdf.

[9] Christine A. Sinsky et al., "'Core Teams': Nurse-Physician Partnerships Provide Patient-Centered Care at an Iowa Practice," *Health Affairs* 29, no. 5 (2010): 966-968.

[10] Michael Kanter et al., "Proactive Office Encounter"; Truls Østbye et al., "Is There Time for Management of Patients with Chronic Diseases in Primary Care?"; Kimberly S. H. Yarnall et al., "Primary Care: Is There Enough Time for Prevention?"

[11] Susan Albers Mohrman, Susan G. Cohen, and Allan M. Mohrman, Jr., *Designing Team-Based Organizations: New Forms for Knowledge Work* (San Francisco: Jossey-Bass, 1995).

[12] "UBT Basics," Labor Management Partnership - Coalition of Kaiser Permanente Unions + Kaiser Permanente, 2012, http://www.lmpartnership.org/ubt.

[13] Alliance of Community Health Plans, *Investing in Outcomes, Creating Value*.

[14] Brent C. James and Lucy A. Savitz, "How Intermountain Trimmed Health Care Costs Through Robust Quality Improvement Efforts," *Health Affairs* 30, no. 6 (2011): 1185-1191.

[15] Boel Andersson-Gäre and Duncan Neuhauser, "The Health Care Quality Journey of Jönköping County Council, Sweden," Q Manage Health Care 16, no. 1 (2007): 2-9; T. Bodenheimer, Mats Bojestig, and Goran Henriks, "Making Systemwide Improvements in Health Care: Lessons from Jönköping County, Sweden," *Q Manage Health Care* 16, no. 1 (2007): 10-15.

[16] Ronald Loo, Joel Whittaker, and Violeta Rabrenivich, "National Practice Recommendations for Hematuria: How to Evaluate in the Absence of Strong Evidence?" *The Permanente Journal* 13, no. 1 (2009): 37.

[17] Howard Jung et al., "Association of Hematuria on Microscopic Urinalysis and Risk of Urinary Tract Cancer," *Journal of Urology* 185 (May 2011): 1699.

[18] Jung et al., "Association of Hematuria on Microscopic Urinalysis and Risk of Urinary Tract Cancer."

[19] Loo, Whittaker, and Rabrenivich, "National Practice Recommendations for Hematuria."

[20] Rita F. Redberg, "Cancer Risks and Radiation Exposure From Computed Tomographic Scans: How Can We Be Sure that the Benefits Outweigh the Risks?" *Archives of Internal Medicine* 169, no. 22 (2009): 2049-2050, http://archinte.ama-assn.org/cgi/content/full/169/22/2049?maxtoshow=&hits=10&RESULTFORMAT=&fulltext=overuse+CT+scans&searchid=1&FIRSTINDEX=0&resourcetype=HWCIT#REF-IED90030-2.

[21] Amy Berrington de González et al., "Projected Cancer Risks from Computed Tomographic Scans Performed in the United States in 2007," *Archives of Internal Medicine* 169, no. 22 (2009): 2071-2077, http://archinte.ama-assn.org/cgi/content/abstract/169/22/2071?ijkey=45e6d79523961652c2d366492e773a86a58e3913&keytype2=tf_ipsecsha.

[22] William R. Hendee et al., "Addressing Overutilization in Medical Imaging," *Radiology* 257 (October 2010): 240-245, http://radiology.rsna.org/content/257/1/240.full?sid=a9ea7752-595c-474c-831f-0f3509ac97ac.

[23] Jessica Zigmond, "Explosion in Scan Rates," *Modern Healthcare* 40, no. 8 (2010): 12.

CHAPTER 9 ENDNOTES

[1] Stephen M. Shortell, Lawrence P. Casalino, and Elliott S. Fisher, "Achieving the Vision: Structural Change," in *Partners in Health: How Physicians and Hospitals Can Be Accountable Together*, ed. Francis J. Crosson and Laura A. Tollen (San Francisco: Jossey-Bass, 2010), 46-71.

[2] Cleveland Clinic, *Facts and Figures* (November 23, 2010), http://my.clevelandclinic.org/Documents/About/facts-figures-2010.pdf.

[3] Phillip Longman, *Best Care Anywhere: Why VA Health Care is Better than Yours* (San Francisco: Polipoint Press, 2007).

[4] Susan Albers Mohrman and Arienne McCracken, "A Physician Turned Leader Commits to Building an Award Winning Organization," in *Lessons in Leadership: Learning from Real World Cases*, ed. Donald D. Warrick and Jens Mueller (Chicago: Rossi - Smith, 2011).

[5] "Course Offerings," Institute for Health Care Delivery Research, 2012, http://intermountainhealthcare.org/qualityandresearch/institute/courses/Pages/home.aspx.

[6] Michael L. Tushman and Charles A. O'Reilly III, *Winning Through Innovation: A Practical Guide to Leading Organizational Change and Renewal* (Boston: Harvard Business School Publishing, 2002).